USE THIS
FOR THAT!

YOUR EASY
ESSENTIAL OIL GUIDEBOOK

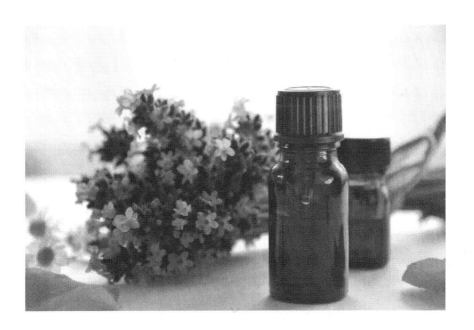

By Kathy Heshelow,
Amazon Best Selling Author; Member, NAHA

(National Association for Holistic Aromatherapy)

Use This For That! Your Easy Essential Oil Guidebook
Text copyright ® 2017 by Kathy Heshelow

Paperback ISBN-13: 978-1548100322
Paperback ISBN-10: 1548100323

Published by Sublime Beauty Naturals®
11125 Park Blvd, Suite 104-103, Seminole FL 33772

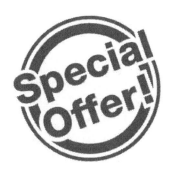

ONCE YOU READ THIS MANUAL, YOU MAY WANT
TO TRY SOME ESSENTIAL OILS. GET 50% YOUR
FIRST PURCHASE OF OUR THERAPEUTIC-GRADE
ESSENTIAL OILS

+ SAFETY TIPS + SECRET STUFF

https://goo.gl/qC5FyF

Enjoy! Kathy Heshelow

HOW IS THE BOOK ARRANGED, AND HOW CAN YOU BEST USE IT?

This book is especially meant for those who are new to essential oils and are not sure what to do with them! It's also helpful for those whom are interested but relatively inexperienced, or for those with some experience but need more ideas or guidance! I present the material in several easy ways, with a slightly different approach than with other guides.

The **first chapter** shares a short introductory overview of what essential oils and aromatherapy are, with some important points on using them.

The second chapter of the book focuses on 13 essential oils which are among the most common and well-used today. I apply the book theme, **"USE THIS FOR THAT"** and show how you can use each one of these popular essential oils and for what purposes. If you are new to essential oils, you may be surprised at the variety of uses possible for just one essential oil. This is thanks to the components and complex makeup of each essential oil, and is one of the reasons I say they have "super powers".

This particular section of the book keeps things simple! You will come away with an understanding of how you can **"USE THIS FOR THAT."**

The third chapter of the book looks at things from the specific issues you may have (stress, insomnia, cuts or burns, colds or coughs, immune system, depression, indigestion, etc.) and shares various essential oils, recipes, research, techniques and suggestions which could be helpful.

4

In other words, if you are experiencing issues with insomnia and want to find some applications that might help, you can refer to the third part of the book by specific issue. You will learn how to **"USE THIS FOR THAT"** by issue. I also include my personal favorites in this section.

By the way, there will be far more essential oils mentioned in this section that just the thirteen I highlighted in the second section of the book!

At the end, I make some recommendations for your "Essential Oil Home Pharmacy", and link to a podcast I did on the subject. I also include a chart and information on Dosages & Dilutions.

Everyone should pay attention to the **Safety Tips** near the beginning of the book, and review them before proceeding to try essential oils. I also send the list as a helpful download if you opt in at the beginning of the book.

Essential oils are relatively safe and natural products – but remember, poison ivy is a "natural plant" but look what it can do! There are some basics you should understand before you use them. Especially do take caution with small children.

To your happiness and wellness! Kathy Heshelow

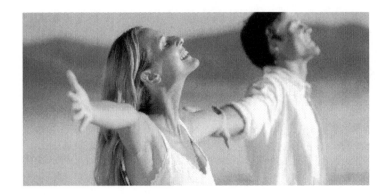

FDA & Disclaimer Statement

The official FDA disclaimer: "These statements have not been evaluated by the Food and Drug Administration. These products are not intended to diagnose, treat, cure, or prevent disease."

Essential Oils and aromatherapy, for me, support what the body needs and requires to thrive, they work at the holistic level of mind-body-spirit, and are time-tested through the centuries.

I fully stand behind the natural wellness properties of Essential Oils, using them in my daily life. However, the statements in this book are not intended as a substitute for professional healthcare nor meant to diagnose, cure or prevent medical conditions or serious disease.

TABLE OF CONTENTS

SAFETY TIPS!

Because this handbook is about suggestions for common wellness problems, it is imperative to understand the safety tips!

Essential oils are pure, plant-based extracted liquids that hold special powers. They are generally known to be safe BUT there are safety precautions to understand.

This is not a definitive list, but I cover the biggest issues. Understand that while essential oils are beneficial and natural, there are some cautions.

It is very hard to overdose on essential oils when using them topically or by inhaling, and most essential oils do not cause side effects like some traditional medicines can. However, we have listed key safety points for you here:

1. **CHILDREN:** If you have young children, PLEASE keep essential oils in a locked cabinet or away from easy access. Young children can be fascinated with the look and smell of essential oils. If accidental ingestion occurs, contact poison control immediately.

2. **EYES:** Keep essential oils away from your eyes! If you get essential oils in your eyes, irrigate with a sterile saline solution or a vegetable oil for 15 minutes. Immediately consult a physician if pain persists after the eye wash.

3. **DILUTE FOR SKIN:** A good rule of thumb is to never use a pure single essential oil undiluted directly on skin, also called using it "neat". (Single oils are diffused in a diffuser, inhaled

12

from the bottle or another device, or mixed with a carrier oil to be used topically. More on carrier oils in Chapter 1.) Exceptions can be made for Lavender, Rose Geranium, Frankincense and perhaps Tea Tree Essential Oil (and any others mentioned in the book), but only after a patch test on your skin.

4. **PATCH TEST:** I like to recommend a small skin patch test prior to every first-time use of an essential oil or essential oil blend, to be safe (especially if you have sensitive skin or health issues.) If any reaction occurs, use plentiful soap and water (or milk!) on the patch area and rinse well. (Reactions are not common.)

5. **FLAMMABLE:** Essential oils are highly flammable; use extreme care around fire.

6. **INGESTION ISSUES:** In general, essential oils are NOT ingested. Some oils can be toxic if ingested even in small amounts. They should only be taken internally under the supervision of a licensed medical practitioner. <u>Keep in mind, the use of essential oils is called</u> **AROMA**<u>therapy.</u>

<u>**The highest and best use, plus fastest and most effective is by inhalation, with the immediate interaction in the brain & control center of your body.**</u>

Some essential oils are good for topical use (diluted in a carrier oil) such as for burns, cuts, headaches, indigestion, inflammation…When or if ingested, essential oils will be broken down by your digestive juices, liver and kidney and may not even be used by the body for its intended purpose – but certain oils could cause serious harm, from internal burns to poisoning.

Essential oils are HIGHLY CONCENTRATED and can burn mucosa or interact in the body (remember #3 and #4 regarding your skin on the list above). So stick with a certified aromatherapist if ingestion is considered for an ailment. Don't experiment.

7. **LOWER DOSES:** Babies, pets and the elderly (especially those weaker in health) require lower doses of essential oils, half that recommended for a healthy adult. In fact, take caution with very young babies; take care with certain essential oils under the age of 5 like Eucalptus, Oregano or Peppermint, and only specific essential oils are recommended for pets (see below.) See our Dosage Chart at the end of the book.

8. **ASTHMA & EPILEPSY PATIENTS:** Asthma and epilepsy patients should avoid Fennel, Hyssop and Rosemary – and in our opinion, asthma sufferers should proceed with caution in general when introducing new essential oils into their environment or body. Some could be helpful indeed, but asthma sufferers could be more sensitive and susceptible. Refer to your certified aromatherapist or doctor.

9. **CANCER PATIENTS**: Cancer patients may use mild dilutions of Bergamot, Chamomile, Lavender, Ginger and/or Frankincense (check with your doctor, aromatherapist or holistic doctor); for nausea, Peppermint may be considered. Note that Fennel and Aniseed in particular should be avoided. Just before and while undergoing chemotherapy essential oils should be

14

avoided unless prescribed by a licensed or certified practitioner (as it could impede chemo action.) It is more common to use them after chemo for something like nausea or calmness.

10. **HIGH BLOOD PRESSURE?** High blood pressure patients should avoid Black Pepper, Clove, Hyssop, Peppermint, Rosemary, Sage and Thyme Essential Oils.

11. **LOW BLOOD PRESSURE?** Low blood pressure patients should avoid excessive use of Lavender.

12. **KIDNEY PROBLEMS?** Sufferers of kidney problems should be cautious if they use Juniper, Sandalwood, or Coriander.

13. **DAILY ASPIRIN USERS**: Methyl salicylate is the active ingredient in aspirin as well as Sweet Birch and Wintergreen Essential Oils. If you use aspirin for medicinal purposes you should avoid these two essential oils due to the risk of overdose.

14. **BLOOD THINNING MEDS**: Clove, Thyme and Oregano Essential Oils (and any excessive use of Turmeric) should be avoided by people taking anticoagulant medication, with clotting or bleeding disorders, major surgery, childbirth, peptic ulcer or hemophilia. These essential oils "thin" the blood and could cause excessive bleeding.

15. **PHOTO-TOXIC (SUN INTERACTION)**: Angelica, Bergamot and ALL of the Citrus Oils (i.e. Lemon, Orange, Grapefruit, Tangerine, Lime, etc.) are photo-toxic. Do not use these oils in skincare blends topically (mixed into shea butter, lotions, serums) if going into the sun or using a tanning bed.

Inhaling or diffusing is no problem for use while being in the sun.

16. **PREGNANT?** Pregnant women should avoid essential oils before the 18th week of pregnancy, especially in cases of prior miscarriage. In the second trimester, essential oils may possibly be used in low doses ONLY if formulated by a professional aromatherapist or health care provider. In our opinion, to be safe, wait until the third trimester or consult a doctor or certified aromatherapist – or wait until the baby is born.

SPECIAL WARNING FOR CAT & DOG OWNERS

Some essential oils can be toxic for cats, and a few for dogs. Kitties have a very acute sense of smell, and they absorb essential oils fast due to a thin skin layer. Unfortunately, they cannot metabolize certain compounds in certain essential oils and so the oils could build up in the system. (Cats are especially susceptible to phenols and ketones.)

We do not recommend using essential oils directly or diluted on your cat. If you are diffusing, be sure to have an open space and a way for the cat to leave the room and get away from diffusing essential oils if they need to.

Dogs may be able to tolerate essential oils but in small diffusions and if applying, NEVER apply to the nose, ears, anus, genitals or use for ingestion.

Here are specifics courtesy of Annares Natural Health:

A List of Some Essential Oils that are Known to be Toxic to Cats:

- Peppermint
- Oregano
- Clove
- Lemon, Orange, Bergamot and all citrus oils
- Melaleuca (tea tree oil)
- Cinnamon (and cassia)
- Wintergreen
- Thyme
- Birch
- Pine
- Spruce
- Any other oils containing phenols

Examples of oils containing Phenols – Wintergreen, Anise, Birch, Clove, Basil, Tarragon, Fennel, Oregano, Thyme, Mountain Savory, Peppermint, Tea Tree, Calamus, Cinnamon Bark, Citronella, Marjoram, Nutmeg, Eucalyptus, Parsley, Ylang Ylang. These all contain greater than 8% phenols.

Some Essential Oils Considered Generally SAFE Around Cats:

- Clary Sage Essential Oil
- Elemi Essential Oil
- Frankincense Essential Oil
- Geranium (Rose Geranium) Essential Oil
- Helichrysum Essential Oil
- Balsam Fir Essential Oil

- Lavender Essential Oil
- Roman Chamomile Essential Oil
- Rosemary Essential Oil

Please refer to a knowledgeable vet or certified aromatherapist when using essential oils around or for your pets. **There are several good books specializing in this on Amazon.**

Chapter 1

OVERVIEW OF ESSENTIAL OILS & AROMATHERAPY

Essential oils are the concentrated aromatic essences extracted from certain plants. They are sometimes called the "life force" or "soul" of a plant, or the "plant's physician" – and they have wonderful powers.

Essential oils are extracted from the flower, leaf, bark, twig, peel, root or other parts (depending on the plant), and method of extraction is typically steam distillation or cold press (though there are a few other methods as well.)

They are complex! Each essential oil will contain many different chemical compounds and constituents, each of which holds specific therapeutic property.

Virtually all essential oils are anti-bacterial (to varying degrees) and some are also anti-fungal and anti-viral!

I wrote about the complexity in the books "The Crisis of Antibiotic-Resistant Bacteria and How Essential Oils Help" and "Essential Oils Have Super Powers" if you want to go deeper into the subject. Just understand, it is this very complexity of essential oils that overcomes and kills bacteria and microbes where antibiotics are failing.

This complexity of composition also allows each specific essential oil to do many different things. It gives them versatility!

Depending on its chemical composition, each essential oil will excel in certain areas.

Essential oils are used in aromatherapy for physical actions as well as emotional balance & wellness. I will refer to both in the book – for instance, help with inflammation or a burn as well as stress or depression.

In this book, I refer to using pure therapeutic-grade essential oils extracted from plants (not synthetic oils or perfumes). They can be used singly (like Lavender or Frankincense) or in blends (like the DeStress blend or blend of your own making.)

HERE ARE JUST A FEW THINGS ESSENTIAL OILS CAN DO:

* KILL BACTERIA, VIRUSES AND FUNGI;

* BRING DOWN INFLAMMATION;

* HELP WITH SLEEP, RELAXATION & STRESS;

* REDUCE CONGESTION & HELP CALM COUGHS;

* REDUCE NAUSEA, INDIGESTION, IBS, CRAMPS;

* HELP HEAL CUTS & BURNS;

* HELP BRING DOWN FEVER;

* HELP REDUCE OR CHASE AWAY HEADACHES;

* HELP SUPPORT YOUR IMMUNE SYSTEM;

* and UPLIFT YOUR MOOD, BRING FOCUS, TRANQUILITY, HELP WITH MEMORY & MORE.

Essential oils are used for mind, body and spirit! And on top of everything else, most of them smell amazing and are enjoyable to use!

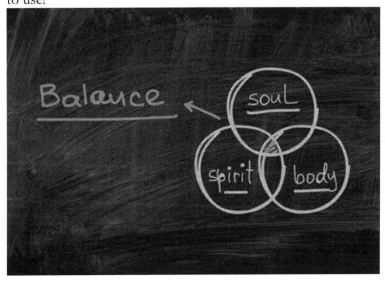

You will discover ways to use them for preventative care (like keeping your immune system strong) and active care (like reducing headache or bringing down a fever).

Essential oils accomplish this for the most part without side effects that some typical pharmaceuticals may have (many pharmaceuticals in fact try to copy plants and their powers.)

Drugs, especially antibiotics, and toxins may kill good flora in the gut or body thereby lowering our level of health or ability to stay balanced, or create unwanted side effects. Essential oils do not typically create these side effects, and they certainly do not kill good flora – they help them!

HOW DO ESSENTIAL OILS ENTER THE BODY AND WORK

There are three ways for Essential Oils to enter your body and conduct their magic:

1) **Inhalation through the nose to the brain and limbic system** (and then dispersed in your body through the lungs and into the bloodstream)

2) **Absorption through the skin** when topically applied, and to the bloodstream for further delivery

3) Internal ingestion (not typically used in the U.S., not recommended in this book and not recommended without professional supervision). Remember, this is called **aroma**therapy.

YOUR LIMBIC SYSTEM IS YOUR DASHBOARD CONTROL CENTER IN THE BRAIN

Your sense of smell is the ONLY one of the five senses tied directly to the limbic system in your brain. This is the <u>oldest area of the brain</u> which deals with emotional and psychological responses.

<u>The limbic system is like your own personal dashboard</u> or control panel: it controls memory and formation of memories, emotion, sex drive, sleep cycles, thirst and physiological actions (like heart rate and breathing rate), time perception, instincts and

motivation.

When the limbic system is activated by scent, a reaction occurs – from calming to invigorating, from secretion of certain hormones or changing body systems (such as slowing the heart rate in an anxiety attack) - and the reaction occurs immediately.

Scent is tied to emotions and intelligence as well as memory. Think of how you react or feel when you smell fresh rain or grass being cut, a fresh Christmas tree, the perfume your mother wore, or the scent of your school gym. Also see how you react to rancid meat – it is a protective action that keeps you from eating it and becoming sick.

Some essential oils like Rosemary bring down the cortisol level which can help calm us during anxiety (when cortisol levels shoot up), while others are stimulating like Eucalyptus or Lemon.

HOW WILL I <u>USE</u> ESSENTIAL OILS?

1] **INHALATION** – typically accomplished with diffusers, inhalers, aromatherapy jewelry, a steam tent or simply inhaling from the bottle!

Most essential oils are lovely to diffuse at home, to clarify and purify the air of microbes but also to add atmosphere (based on what the particular essential oil can do). So if you need to bring the energy of the home to one of tranquility in the evening hours, for instance, Frankincense or Lavender are good choices. If you suffer from insomnia, diffusing Lavender in your bedroom can do wonders. If you need help with focus or uplift, you could diffuse Bergamot, Sweet Orange, Neroli, Peppermint or Basil, to name a few.

You can just breathe in from the bottle, or use an inhaler. Even an essential oil on a tissue or cotton ball sometimes suffices.

You can put a few drops on a <u>lava stone bracelet</u> or aromatherapy necklace and pull the jewelry to your nose when you wish to inhale more intensely during the day.

If suffering from a cold, sinus infection or cough, you might do a steam tent over a bowl as a proactive treatment, inhaling the essential oil(s).

2] **TOPICAL APPLICATION** – typically you can purchase a blend already made for you, make you own by mixing the chosen oils into a cream, gel or oil; use on a compress; use in a bath; and a very few can be applied directly to skin (called "neat".)

Using essential oils topically can help very specific issues: for instance, to bring the inflammation of a swollen or sprained ankle, disinfect a cut, to gain relief from a headache, improve skin by using essential oils in a facial cream, or bring down indigestion by massaging a blend on your tummy.

As mentioned previously, in a few exceptional cases, an essential oil could be applied directly to your skin without a carrier oil (such as Lavender on a cut, but only after a patch test.)

You might use essential oils in a bath (or on bath crystals or salts) or in a foot soak so that you will not only inhale the scent but absorb them through your skin.

BASIC TOOLS TO USE

DIFFUSER: For diffusing essential oils into the air where you can breathe them, you use a diffuser! There are several different types. The most used and popular today are ultrasonic diffusers with a water container that create a mist diffusion. You put drops of your essential oil or oils into the water container, turn it on, and you are diffusing in a matter of seconds!

We recommend to always buy one with an auto-stop feature (if the water runs low, it stops). All have a "continuous run" feature, but many have features such as "on one minute, off one minute cycles" which are helpful for overnight diffusion. Some light up with LED lights or are quite decorative, while others are just functional. There are many choices, and you can find selections on Amazon.

Another type of diffuser is the nebulizer. This one does not use water – it diffuses the essential oil(s) directly. It is more pure, and helpful if you don't want humidity in the air, but they are messier and take more maintenance.

Older style diffusion is/was a candle underneath a cup of water. Many don't use these anymore because of the fire hazard and they aren't as effective as a mister.

STEAM TENT. This is what it sounds like. You boil water, then add your drops of essential oils, and cover your head with a towel or large cloth and breathe in the steam & oils. This is good when you have a cold, sinus problems, some skin issues, coughs, etc. as described in the book.

INHALERS are mentioned throughout the book. These are simple little devices whereby you add your essential oil(s) to cotton or a filler inside the device, and then you can take it with you on the go. It is great on an airplane, for instance, where you can't diffuse, in the metro or train, in the office, at the movies or out and about!

You can certainly take a bottle of your essential oil with you on the go and inhale from it, but using an inhaler will protect your bottle and precious essential oil longer. You won't be exposing it to heat, light, or opening it as often for oxidation to occur. Using 10 or 15 drops in an inhaler, which will last for months, seems a better way to do it.

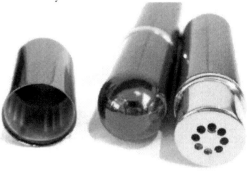

AROMATHERAPY JEWELRY is a fun way to have your essential oils near you all day. You put a drop on your lava stone bracelet or necklace filler.

CARRIER OILS

This is simply the term used for the oil (or gel or cream) in which you will blend drops of your essential oil or oils for topical use. Remember, most essential oils are very powerful and concentrated and can agitate the skin if used directly.

Using a carrier allows for topical use, and it helps "carry" the essential oil into your system. They are also helpful in their own right, depending on the oil, for specific issues!

Jojoba is always a good choice for all skin types, as it is close to our skin's sebum, has a long shelf live and is stable as well as nourishing.

Dry skin loves Avocado, Almond, Sesame, Jojoba, and Baobab (full of vitamins and minerals.

Normal skin loves Apricot, Almond, Avocado, Jojoba, Baobab, Safflower and Carrot Seed.

Oily skin loves Jojoba!

You may want to use a cream for something like anti-aging or dry skin facial creams, or a gel for something like a burn or hand-sanitizer. Oils are the best carriers for essential oils, but other modes can work, depending on the application and your desires!

BIOAVAILABILITY and HALF-LIFE OF ESSENTIAL OILS

These are important concepts to understand in your use of essential oils. Bioavailability refers to the amount of the essential oil that is taken in and used by the body. Half-life, also called "peak concession", is the amount of time that the essential oil is used by the body for effectiveness.

See the outline on the next page to get a grasp of this concept! You can listen to **my short podcast** (Essential Oil Zen) which explains this if you process information better that way!

THE BOTTOM LINE? Inhalation is the fastest and most effective use of essential oils. Topical application has slower but longer use by your body and is not as bioavailable, but is effective for such things as cuts, burns or compresses.

Finally, if you are going to do a few of your own blends, refer to our **DOSAGE CHART** recommendations at the back of the book. This helps understand the amounts of the essential oil you should blend into your carrier depending on the situation and health of the recipient.

Always check with a doctor, holistic or integrative doctor or aromatherapist if you are on medications or suffering from a serious disease. You may consider buying pre-made blends if blending is beyond your interest, time or scope.

Take a look at the Bioavailability chart on the next page, and then let's get to the meat of "Use This for That!"

In general, **the only 100% Bioavailability is when a substance is injected.**

ESSENTIAL OILS:
+ INHALED: Bioavailability can be 70%

+ Compare this to an oral drug like morphine with only 23.9% bioavailability
(Any drug swallowed, that goes through the stomach and processed by the liver typically has a lower bioavailability)

+ TOPICAL:
Bioavailability is generally about 7-9%.

HALF-LIFE
Also called "peak concession"
(that is, when half of the essential oil has reached its EFFECTIVE PEAK and will start to wane):

+ TOPICAL – peak concession is 360 minutes
+ INHALED – peak concession is 20 minutes

Chapter 2

USE THIS FOR THAT!

13 MOST COMMON, VERSATILE AND USEFUL ESSENTIAL OILS, & WHAT THEY CAN DO FOR YOU

As mentioned in the preface, this chapter will focus on 13 wonderful, popular, versatile and most basic essential oils. There are hundreds of essential oils, but in this section, I focus on those that can serve you well. You will understand key basics that each can assist you and your family with.

They are:

Lavender	Clary Sage
Frankincense	Bergamot
Eucalyptus	Rose Geranium
Lemon	Cedarwood
Rosemary	Tea Tree
Peppermint	Turmeric

Clove Bud

Lavender

Use This – <u>LAVENDER</u> - For That:

Use this for INSOMNIA

Use this for CUTS OR BURNS

Use this for STRESS OR ANXIETY

Use this for INFLAMMATION AND PAIN

Use this for SCORPIONS, PESTS & INSECT BITES

Use this for FRESHENING OF AIR OR LAUNDRY

Use this for IMMUNE SUPPORT

Latin Name: Lavendula Augustifolia Steam Distilled (Flowers)

Lavender is high in the constituent linalol, which gives it excellent analgesic qualities.

INSOMNIA: Lavender is the best essential oil for insomnia and sleep problems. It is soothing, relaxing and clinical tests show it could help you reach deeper levels of sleep.

The best way to use it for insomnia is to diffuse it in the bedroom.

Be sure your diffuser has the "auto stop" feature (when water runs low, it stops); if the settings include one that is on for a minute/off for a minute, it lasts longer through the night and works well.

If you are unable to diffuse Lavender (perhaps a partner doesn't like the scent), you can put an inhaler under your pillow. Take 3 or 4 deep breathes when you lay down to sleep, and use again as you need.

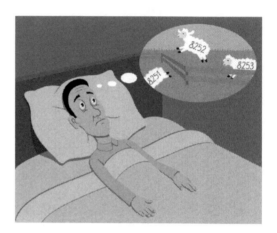

You could also dot some Lavender on your wrist and under your nostrils, and breathe in. In addition, you could put 10 drops in an ounce of cream and massage some on your temples, neck and wrist at night. Remember bioavailability – inhaling will do the best and fastest work, but topical will also help.

CUTS & BURNS: Lavender is one of the few essential oils you can use "neat", that is, directly on your skin without blending it in a carrier oil or cream. (However, do a patch test to be sure there is no irritation for you, long before you would need to use it for a cut or burn.)

Lavender, like all essential oils, holds strong antibacterial powers and is good to disinfect a cut or burn; and to start the healing process. A few drops on your cut or burn will help you right away.

Lavender is actually infamous because of the modern-era "father of aromatherapy", Rene-Maurice Gattefosse. He was a chemist for a prominent perfumer, working in the south of France, and one day received a horrific burn on his arm in the lab following an accident.

He extinguished the fire by rolling in the grass but gas gangrene was rapidly developing (gas gangrene is life threatening.) He rinsed his arm with Lavender Essential Oil, which stopped the gasification, and eventually healed him very well. In addition, other burns and blisters he had from previous accidents were also healed. This set him on a lifelong path of discovery and passion for essential oils, and he devoted his entire life to its study!

By the way, Gattefosse is the one who termed the industry "aromatherapie" or aromatherapy in English, to describe the healing process with essential oils!

STRESS or ANXIETY: Lavender is a wonderful essential oil to help bring down stress levels or anxiety.

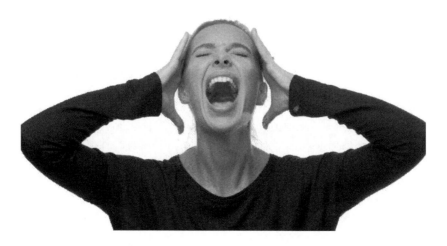

Inhale it at once if you are stressed or feel anxious; or diffuse it. You can inhale it from the bottle; use an inhaler if you are on the move. Aromatherapy jewelry could serve you well, too.

If you suffer from chronic stress or even anger, in addition to inhaling when you feel the emotion coming on, consider using some Lavender in your body cream or oil, in your soaps or shampoo.

Lavender is one of the essential oils being used in the treatment of returning war vets who suffer PTSD or anxiety, and in more and more hospital settings. It is also helping cancer patients or those in the hospital who have high stress levels or those finding it hard to sleep in the hospital.

Relaxing Foot Massage: Add 10 drops of Lavender to 1 ounce of a carrier oil; massage (or have someone massage) your feet and let the goodness absorb!

INFLAMMATION: Lavender is an analgesic and can help reduce pain levels (including for cuts and burns).

For a swollen or sprained ankle, arms or achy muscles: Do a cold compress. Put 5-6 drops of Lavender and 2 drops Frankincense in a bowl of water, soak the compress (like a washcloth) in it, and then wring it out and place on the affected area.

For inflammation like arthritis, put drops in a cream or body oil, and massage into your skin daily. You could put 4 drops lavender and 5 drops Frankincense (+ 2 drops of Turmeric if you like).

SCORPIONS, PESTS and INSECT BITES: In hot climates, scorpions may want to come in the house. Scorpions HATE Lavender (as people in the south of France well know!) Put drops on the windowsill or around the door area to help repel them! Put them on cotton balls or teabags and slip inside cabinets, drawers or corners. Lavender cuttings do the same thing!

Want to repel insects from your body? Add some Lavender to your body cream or oil and massage it in. Unlike citrus oils (which are known as pest repellents but sun-toxic), there is no problem in the sun with Lavender. This isn't like using DEET, or course, but can be helpful.

(P.S. A few other non-citrus essential oils could also do the trick of repelling pests, like Peppermint, Clove bud and Cedarwood.)

Bug bite that hurts or itches? Put 2 drops of Lavender on it "neat" directly several times daily to help reduce itching and swelling. (Peppermint is also good for this purpose.)

5

FRESHEN THE AIR OR LAUNDRY: Diffuse Lavender at home to freshen the air as well as kill microbes.

Put 1-2 drops in your washer and in your dishwasher for a little freshening up and antibacterial work. You could also put a few drops on a cloth and place in your dryer. Using essential ils in this way after someone has the cold or flu can be helpful, too.

BONUS – ANTIBACTERIAL: Remember, virtually all essential oils have anti-bacterial power (some are stronger than others, of course, depending on their components.)

Note that researchers at Cornell University found that Lavender oil can eradicate certain antibiotic-resistant bacteria, including more than one strain of pathogenic Staphylococcus and pathogenic Streptococcus (often involved in coughs and colds.)

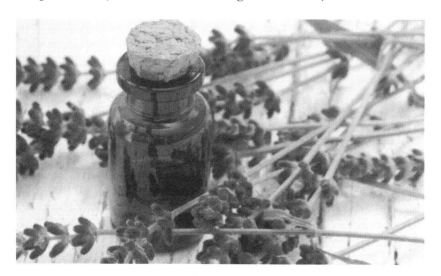

Frankincense

Use This – <u>FRANKINCENSE</u> – For That:

Use This For TRANQUILITY and MINDFULNESS

Use This for CELL REGENERATION

Use This for INFLAMMATION

Use This for ONGOING RESPIRATORY ISSUES

Use This to BOOST IMMUNITY

Latin Name: Boswellia Carterii Resin from Tree is Steam Distilled

TRANQUILITY: Frankincense is lovely for tranquility, relaxation and quiet focus. It's great to use for meditation, after exercising (with the added bonus of anti-inflammation), or at home in the evening. I love to diffuse it in the office when I am writing – it simply makes me feel good.

CELL REGENERATION: Frankincense is known for powers of cell regeneration – hence it can be a great anti-aging tonic or for use in your beauty products. Put some drops (about 5-6 drops per ounce) in your facial cream or body oil. Because it is also an anti-inflammatory, you'll get double benefits.

ONGOING RESPIRATORY ISSUES: While we tend to think of Eucalyptus first, if you have chronic ongoing respiratory issues, you could benefit from using Frankincense on a regular basis in different formats: drops in an oil or cream massaged on your chest, a drop to your shampoo, inhaled from a diffuser, or several drops in a bath or foot soak. It can also help with a temporary build-up of phlegm – use 3-5 drops in your cream or oil and massage on the throat, chest and even temples.

INFLAMMATION: If you suffer from arthritis or rheumatoid arthritis, consider incorporating Frankincense into your products (along with Turmeric).

In the U.K., Cardiff University scientists found that Frankincense could inhibit the production of key inflammatory molecules, helping prevent the breakdown of the cartilage tissue that causes these conditions. (ScienceDaily August 4, 2011.) Put 6-10 drops of Frankincense in an oil or organic cream, and rub topically on hands or joints daily or 4 times weekly.

BOOST IMMUNITY: Part of having a healthy and efficient immune system is the regulation of inflammation. Frankincense helps with this, in addition to its general abilities and promoting of tranquility.

There are serious ongoing studies about Frankincense and cancer prevention, including brain cancer, but the studies have further to go.

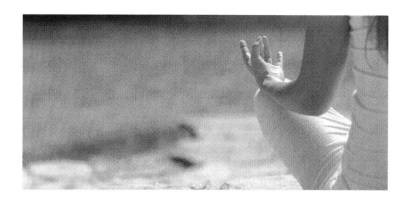

Clove Bud

Use This – <u>CLOVE BUD</u> – For That

Use This for a Strong BACTERICIDE

Use This to Stimulate the IMMUNE SYSTEM

Use This for ORAL CARE

Use This to WARM AND BRIGHTEN, PROVIDE EMOTIONAL SUPPORT

Use This to LOOSEN TIGHT MUSCLES & PAIN

Use This to REPEL BUGS & SPIDERS

Latin Name: Eugenia caryophyllata The flower buds are Steam Distilled

STRONG BACTERICIDE: Clove is one of few essential oils in which no bacteria, virus or fungi can live in its presence. When combined with Lavender, it has additive effects against bacteria.

Clinical tests proved that Clove Bud Essential Oil is effective against HSV I and HSV II (herpes). Clove was one of the essential oils used in a famed French test: 210 petri dish colonies of bacteria, fungi and viruses were bred, and then essential oils were diffused in the room. After 15 minutes of diffusion, all but 14 colonies were dead, and <u>everything was dead after 30 minutes</u>.

Diffuse Clove, or use it in your inhaler – I do often. I love to use Clove Bud and Eucalyptus together in an inhaler when I travel in bacteria-prone airplanes!

STIMULATE AND SUPPORT THE IMMUNE SYSTEM:
Clove Bud can help stimulate the immune system, and support its
function. Include in your diffuser, or incorporate into your body
creams.

ORAL CARE: First, do NOT put Clove directly in your mouth –
it is quite strong and could burn you. Clove can be used in your
organic oil for Oil Pulling to kill bacteria and viruses (put 3 drops in
a tablespoon of oil, and then swish!) Put some drops in warm
water and swish around your mouth after brushing your teeth. Put
a drop or two on your toothpaste!

Not sure what Oil Pulling is? Read more on my site here. It is an
ancient yet popular method for stellar oral care!

ORAL PAIN: In one study published in The Journal of Dentistry
in 2006 (there have been many other studies), a team of dentists
recruited 73 adult volunteers and randomly split them into groups
that had one of four substances applied to the gums just next to the
canine tooth: a clove gel, benzocaine, a placebo resembling the
clove gel, or a placebo resembling benzocaine. (In this study, Clove
Essential Oil was added to a gel – not used directly.) Then, after
five minutes, they compared what happened when the subjects
received two needle sticks in those areas. Not surprisingly, the
placebos failed to numb the tissue against the pain, but the Clove
and benzocaine applications numbed the tissue equally well. "No
significant difference was observed between Clove and benzocaine
regarding pain scores," the scientists concluded. Clove performs!

TOOTH ACHE? Dip a Q-tip into a little Clove, and touch it on
the affected area. This will help relieve inflammation, be an
antiseptic against bacteria and pain reliever. But please be careful, as

11

Clove is potent!

FEELING DOWN, COLD (EMOTIONAL OR PHYSICAL):
Clove's warmth and brightening qualities are excellent. Diffuse or
inhale; or blend into a carrier for a massage oil.

TIGHT MUSCLES OR PAIN: Tight muscles, bad pain in legs or
shoulders? Clove can help relieve muscular tension and warms plus
boosts circulation. Blend 7-10 drops alone or with a few drops with
Bergamot, Lavender or Rose Geranium into an ounce of carrier oil
or cream and massage into the affected area.

REPEL SPIDERS & BUGS: Many bugs are repelled by Clove!
Simply diffuse, or put some drops on cotton balls or tea bags and
set them where they can repel. Use in a body cream.

SAFETY TIP: As mentioned in the safety tips, remember that
Clove thins the blood so if you are on blood thinners, avoid or use
rarely in very small doses, or consult your doctor

Peppermint

Use This – <u>PEPPERMINT</u> – For That

Use This for INDIGESTION, NAUSEA, IBS

Use This for DIZZINESS & SEASICKNESS

Use This for HAY FEVER and SOME ALLERGIES

Use This for HEADACHES

Use This to REDUCE SUGAR CRAVINGS & LOSE WEIGHT

Use This as a BACTERICIDE (AND ORAL CARE)

Use This For TIRED ACHY FEET

Use This for NEUROPATHIC PAIN, AND POST SHINGLES RECOVERY

Use This for CHILDREN'S HEAD LICE

Use This to REDUCE ACNE or BREAKOUTS

Use This to Repel ANTS OR MICE

Latin name: Mentha piperita Production: Steam Distilled (leaves)

Peppermint is INCREDIBLY versatile, as you can see above. The wide variety of uses makes it very popular and a very useful essential oil.

NAUSEA, UPSET TUMMY, IBS, SEASICKNESS:

Peppermint is very well known for relieving nausea, upset stomach, and vomiting. Inhale Peppermint oil right away when you feel nauseous. It can eliminate the effects of nausea while relaxing and soothing you. Put 3 drops in a tablespoon of an oil or cream, and massage on your forehead or temples and tummy. Be sure to inhale and use topically – both methods (inhaling & topical) give you added coverage in 2 channels of your body systems.

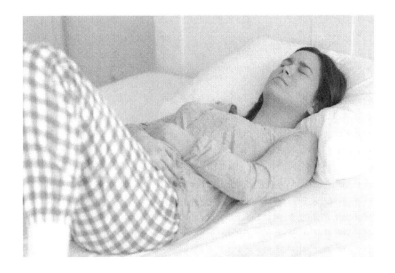

Chemotherapy-Induced Nausea: A 2013 study found that Peppermint oil was found to be effective in reducing chemotherapy-induced nausea, and at reduced cost versus standard drug-based treatment (plus safer and more pleasant – my comments). Some hospitals and clinics now recommend it.

HAY FEVER: Allergic rhinitis (hay fever) could be helped by Peppermint. A 2001 preclinical study found that extracts of the leaves of Peppermint inhibit histamine release indicating it may be clinically effective in alleviating the nasal symptoms of allergic rhinitis. Kill off the offenders in your nasal cavities and purify as well as help with the symptoms.

If hay fever hits, inhale (use in an inhaler, or do a tent steam with 5 drops of peppermint in the hot water. You may add a drop of Eucalyptus if sinuses are already inflamed or you have congestion.) Peppermint helps your respiratory system and will help clear up phlegm or congestion, while helping to reduce the hay fever effects.

Diffuse Peppermint in your home during hay fever season. You may want to put a few drops on your air-conditioning filters.

HEADACHES: Peppermint can help relieve the pain and stress of headaches. Put 7 drops in a small bowl of water, swish your washcloth or compress in the cool water, wring it out and use on your forehead. Keep it out of your eyes, of course!

REDUCE SUGAR CRAVINGS (AND ADDICTION), HELP WITH WEIGHT LOSS: Peppermint, along with a few other essential oils like Grapefruit, strongly helps you quell sugar cravings. Sugar fires up the same addiction center in the brain as heroin, crack and nicotine. Use of certain essential oils, like Peppermint, help you feel you got your "sweet" fill, and help the craving to pass.

I wrote an entire book with action plans and more on the science of this, found here.

Peppermint can also affect the brain's satiety center, which triggers a sensation of fullness after meals. (Some sugars turn off this function, by the way.) Inhale Peppermint, but you can also – in addition – add 7 drops to an ounce of oil or cream, and apply to your temples and wrists; wear it on aromatherapy jewelry.

ANTI-BACTERIAL: Peppermint Essential Oil contains strong qualities of antiviral, antimicrobial and antifungal. Diffuse it at home as preventative or if someone is sick.

This includes applications for antibacterial ORAL CARE! Like Clove, put a drop on your toothpaste or in your organic oil for Oil Pulling. Peppermint has been found to be superior to the mouthwash chemical chlorhexidine inhibiting Streptococcus mutans-driven biofilm formation associated with dental caries (cavities). It also helps reduce bacteria that cause bad breath.

SHINGLES ASSOCIATED PAIN & NEUROPATHIC ISSUES: A 2002 case study found that topical Peppermint oil treatment resulted in a near immediate improvement of shingles associated neuropathic pain symptoms; the therapeutic effects persisted throughout the entire 2 months of follow-up treatment. Blend 6-7 drops in an ounce of a carrier and massage on the body; plus diffuse.

TIRED ACHY FEET: Soak your feet in water with Peppermint drops. The menthol levels in Peppermint will be refreshing as well as a pain reliever, and relieve spasms.

You can also create a refreshing spray for your feet and lower legs – this is especially good in summer. Using a 4 ounce spray bottle,

16

mix 30 drops of Peppermint in 1 teaspoon of vodka then top off the 4 oz. bottle with distilled water. <u>Always shake before use</u> (water and oil will separate, but water is the carrier. Shaking before use mixes it again.) Mist your feet, ankles and lower legs – it is refreshing and helps revive! It could be good in the summer for refreshing your hot feet, too! (Keep this in the fridge.) Do not spray near your eyes.

HEAD LICE? Did your child get head lice? Use 10 Peppermint drops in the shampoo and massage well; then rinse. Repeat again later in the day and every day (or twice daily) as needed. You can also put some drops of Peppermint in the conditioner, and massage it on and let sit for a while before rinsing. Diffuse it at home, too, and in your child's bedroom during the day if they are there - but not at night, as it is a stimulant. I go into more detail with additional tactics in Chapter 3 under "Head Lice".

ACNE: Breakouts, congested skin, oil or acne? Put 4-7 drops of Peppermint in a steaming bowl of water and form a tent with a towel. Steam your face – then rinse with cool water. You could also put 5 drops of Peppermint and 1 drop of Tea Tree in a gel or jojoba oil, and use as a facial tonic.

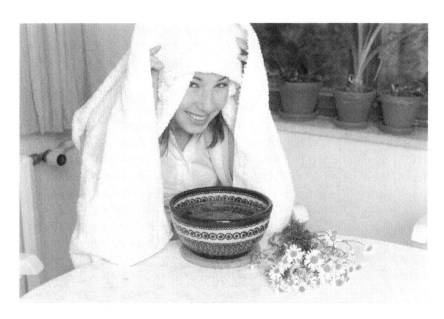

ANTS OR MICE IN THE HOUSE? MOSQUITO BITE OR FIRE ANT BITE? Put 4-5 drops of Peppermint on a tea bag or cotton ball, and place at the back of kitchen cabinets or where there may be holes in the wall or cabinets (points of entry) as a deterrent. Ants and mice especially hate peppermint.

The cooling menthol sensation in Peppermint will help relieve the itch of a mosquito or fire ant bite. Put a drop on direct (after a patch test), or put 7 drops in an ounce of carrier & apply as needed.

Tea Tree

Use This – <u>TEA TREE</u> – For That

Use This for MOLD & FUNGUS

Use This for AN ANTI-BACTERIAL

Use This for ACNE

Use This for ORAL CARE

Use This for SKIN CONDITIONS (LIKE ECZEMA)

Latin name: Melaleuca Alterifolia   Production: Steam Distilled leaves

Tea Tree excels at fungal and mold treatments, but also holds other qualities!

ANTI-BACTERIAL INCLUDING AGAINST MRSA:
Tea Tree was one of the Essential Oils used in a live hospital case to kill MRSA (Methicillin-Resistant Staphylococcus Aureus) also known as an antibiotic-resistant superbug.)

This is reported in my books "Essential Oils Have Super Powers" and in "The Crisis of Antibiotic-Resistant Bacteria and How Essential Oils Can Help." A doctor was able to save a man's leg from amputation, thanks to Tea Tree Essential Oil (and Eucalyptus). The patient had been referred to Dr. Eugene Sherry at the University of Sydney in Australia, after all hope had been lost of

19

stopping a deep MRSA wound. Amputation was being considered. He used a solution of Tea Tree and Eucalyptus on the deep leg wound over a period of 3 weeks and not only killed the MRSA but healed the wound – and the man kept his leg.

Researchers at Australia's Royal Brisbane and Women's Hospital also found that Tea Tree, Eucalyptus and Lemongrass inhibited bacteria in large measure, <u>notably better than rubbing alcohol</u>. They also tested the essential oils against the most deadly of the superbugs and found them to be highly effective.

Diffuse Tea Tree in your home, or use an inhaler. It's good to use in your air conditioning filters to keep mold and fungus out of the ducts. Put some drops on your filter or in the ducts. (If the scent is too medicinal for you, you can add a few drops of Lavender or Rose Geranium to your blend.)

If someone has a nasty cough around you, breathe in tea tree (put some in your inhaler, on a cloth or Kleenex or diffuse if at home) and protect yourself.

FUNGUS & MOLD: Fungus and mold can hide in damp hidden areas of your home (inside of your washing machine liner, the shower corner). Put some Tea Tree on a cloth and wipe down the area. Add a drop of Lemon for extra anti-bacterial action and a touch of freshness. I like to do this in drains, too!

STINKY SHOES: It can also work in stinky shoes! Mix 12 drops Tea Tree in an ounce or so of baking soda (you can also add a few drops of Peppermint or Lavender), sprinkle in your shoes and let them sit overnight; shake them out the next morning.

Tea Tree could help with fungal-based athlete's foot, jock itch and fungal infections of the toenail. <u>However, these issues take a</u>

LONG time to heal, and not everyone has the fortitude to keep up the applications.

a) Athlete's foot – wash your foot or feet thoroughly and make sure they are very dry (fungi and bacteria love moist areas.) Then apply several drops AT LEAST twice per day "neat", unless you have a reaction, and then dilute it in an organic oil or cream. Be consistent, and do this every day until the infection is beat. This can take as long as 6 months if it is a serious infection (same for toenail infection.) As an added measure, you can sprinkle baking soda mixed with tea tree in shoes overnight, then shake it out the next morning.

b) Jock itch – this is a fungal infection. Use drops directly at least twice daily. It will initially help take away the itch, but with time it kills the fungus. One aromatherapist told me that using a few drops of tea tree on the towels and underwear in the washing machine, that is, those in use by the affected person, is also a good practice.

c) Toenail infection – this can be so persistent and long-lasting. Follow the same instructions as for Athlete's foot above, but with a few more cautions. Don't reuse your emery boards or files after a pedicure; do a weekly (at least) foot soak with tea tree oil (add a few drop of Lemon, Clove or Lavender if you wish); disinfect your nail scissors or clippers with tea tree after trimming nails. Be consistent with your applications at least twice daily. It will probably take at least 2 months as the nail will need to grow out fully, but it will be well worth it to show off your feet in summer sandals and at the beach.

ACNE: Tea Tree is known to fight acne, bacteria and oil, and is often found in those types of products. If suffering, do a steam tent with 6-7 drops of Tea Tree to get at the issues; do a tonic or astringent of Tea Tree in witch hazel (6 drops in an ounce); wipe or dab gently with a cotton ball on the affect areas after your steam.

ORAL CARE: Tea Tree is known to fight oral candidiasis, prevent gum disease and help prevent sore throats. Put a drop on your toothpaste, or put a drop in your organic oil for oil pulling to swish in your mouth (I do this from time to time in my Sesame oil, though more often I use Peppermint or Clove). You can also put a few drops in warm water and gargle if you feel a sore throat coming on.

SKIN CONDITIONS LIKE ECZEMA, DERMATITIS OR PSORIASIS? Mix Tea Tree (10 drops), Lavender (5 drops) and baobab oil or coconut oil together (1 ounce) and apply twice daily to skin, or as needed.

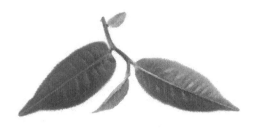

Lemon Essential Oil

Use This – <u>LEMON</u> – For That

Use This for **BETTER CIRCULATION**

Use This to **BRING DOWN FEVER**

Use This for **LIVER PROTECTION & SUPPORT**

Use This to **REDUCE MIGRAINES AND HEADACHES**

Use This for **HOME CLEANING & POLISHING**

Use This to **WASH FRUITS & VEGETABLES**

Use This as a Backup for **NAUSEA**

Use This for **UPLIFT, TO FEEL BRIGHT AND SHARP**

Latin Name: Citrus limon Peels are Cold Pressed

Lemon is a happy, familiar scent to many and beneficial to your wellness – but practical around the house, too!

CIRCULATION: Lemon encourages better circulation! It can help with varicose veins, help with sluggish systems and blocked energy. (This includes helping headaches, too.)

HELP BRING DOWN FEVER: Lemon Essential Oil can help

23

bring down fever and relieve symptoms of flu. (Lemongrass can help with this as well.) Diffuse Lemon; use a cold compress (about 7 drops of lemon up to 10), wring it out and put it on the forehead or body. You could also put it in a cool bath.

LIVER PROTECTION: Lemon Essential Oil offers protection and support of liver functions. An important component in lemon is d-Limonene, and it can increase the rate of synthesis of glutathione S-transferase in the liver. Translation? This is an important enzyme in detoxification and liver protection. Use topically (5 – 7 drops in an ounce of oil, massage on) and inhale.

REDUCE MIGRAINES & HEADACHES: Lemon is one of the essential oils to try for your migraine or headache. Diffuse it or inhale from the bottle (or inhaler.) Do a cold compress and rest in a dark room. Use 6 drops of Lemon in cold water, swish your washcloth or compress in it, ring out and put on your forehead. Do not get Lemon in your eyes!

LEMON FRESH HOME. Lemon Essential Oil can serve as a wood polish, help silver that is tarnished, cleanse hard kitchen and bathroom surfaces. Lemon will cleanse well, and bring fresh uplift to the room while killing bacteria.

a) Surface Cleanser: In large glass spray bottle, mix; 3/4 cup olive oil, 1/4 cup white distilled vinegar, 30-40 drops Lemon essential oil. Shake before using each time (lemon and water separate.) Start in small quantities, wipe down the surface.

b) Wood Polish: Add a few drops to olive oil to clean, protect, buff up and shine wood finishes.

c) Silver Tarnished? Lemon oil is a great remedy for the early stages of tarnish on silver and other metals. But don't use a paper towel – either use a cloth or cotton balls.

d) Fish or another scent from cooking? Diffuse Lemon Essential Oil to clear the air!

FEEL NAUSEOUS? <u>If you don't like Peppermint or don't have any, Lemon can substitute.</u> A recent study showed that symptoms decreased after 2 days in 100 women who suffered nausea and used Lemon Essential Oil. (Inhale deeply, and you can also mix 5-7 drops in an ounce cream and rub on your stomach.)

CLEANSE FRUITS & VEGGIES: Rinse or soak your fruits and vegetables in a gallon of water with 3-5 drops of Lemon Essential Oil. Following a study conducted by the U.S. Department of Agriculture, using Lemon could help protect against such pathogens like E. coli and Salmonella, and can help cleanse toxins from the skin.

BRIGHTEN MOOD, UPLIFT, FOCUS: Diffuse or inhale lemon to brighten your mood, sharpen your sense, bring focus and uplift!

Cedarwood

Use This – <u>CEDARWOOD</u> – For That

Use This for COUGHS, CONGESTION & BRONCHIAL ISSUES

Use This for Various HAIR ISSUES

Use This for IMMUNE SYSTEM SUPPORT

Use This For a REPELLENT

Use This for ORAL CARE

Use This for a METABOLISM STIMULATANT

Use This to FEEL GROUNDED or CONFIDENT

Latin name: Juniperus virginiana or Cupressus Funebris. The bark or bark chips are Steam Distilled

Cedarwood is grounding and earthy, but holds many powers as well. For years, cedarwood chests were popular as they repelled pests.

HAIR LOSS: In France, Cedarwood is included in commercial shampoos and hair lotions for hair loss or alopecia. It can help stimulate the hair follicles and increase circulation to the scalp which can contribute to hair growth and slow hair loss. Herbalists and aromatherapists often recommend it often for this condition.

Some research indicates that Cedarwood blended with Lavender and Rosemary could also help improve hair growth and health, by massaging it in and letting sit for 30 minutes (diluted of course, most often in coconut oil) or adding it to your shampoo. Research shows improvement over a 7 month period with daily use.

DRY SCALP or DANDRUFF. Cedarwood Essential Oil helps reduce dry or flaky skin. It stimulates the scalp and increases circulation (as we saw in the hair loss description.) To take advantage of this essential oil benefit for dandruff or dryness, mix 5 drops of Cedarwood with 1 ounce of coconut oil; massage it on your scalp for five minutes. For the best results, let it sit on your scalp for 30 minutes or so — then wash it out and shampoo as normal.

CHRONIC BRONCHITIS, RESPIRATORY ISSUES & COUGHS. French physicians reported strong results with Cedarwood Essential Oil use in cases of chronic bronchitis. Diffuse it and/or inhale from the bottle or personal inhaler often if suffering. Put 10 drops in an ounce of body cream, gel or oil and massage on your chest, throat, back of neck and wrists.

27

ECZEMA. Eczema is a common skin disorder that causes dry, red, itchy skin that can blister or crack. Cedarwood Essential Oil can help reduce the inflammation that leads to this irritating skin issue; it can help reduce skin peeling. Add 5-10 drops to 1 ounce of your skin lotion, oil or cream and massage on the area; or put 5-10 drops in your bath and have a soak.

ANTISEPTIC: Cedarwood Essential Oil can be applied topically on wounds as an antiseptic (typically blended with coconut oil, an organic gel, or if direct, do your patch test first.) It defends the body against toxins and relieves your white blood cells and immune system of stress or malfunction — this helps protects your internal functions and fights off bacteria in the body. Create a blend by mixing 10 drops of Cedarwood with an ounce of coconut oil, and then rub the mixture on your body to help with wounds or infections.

ASTRINGENT: Add 1-2 drops to your toner for a nice tightening and refreshing feel. You can also do this by adding drops to organic jojoba or an organic aloe gel.

ACNE: Cedarwood is known to help with acne treatment, perhaps not as common as Tea Tree. It helps tighten pores after cleansing them. Use a few drops in a cleanser or as mentioned above, as an astringent. You could also add Cedarwood to coconut oil mixed with oatmeal for a scrub – you might add a few drops of Tea Tree!

INSECT REPELLENT: Cedarwood was originally used in chests and storage boxes thanks to the repellent nature of the wood, to protect contents of the box from critters. It has been found to repel all sorts of insects, including moths and mosquitos. Since citrus essential oils (like Lemongrass and Lemon) are very effective repellents but CANNOT be used on the skin in daytime due to the strong sun-toxic reactions, Cedarwood could be used as a topical option. Add to your cream (5-7 drops in an ounce), or put 5-7 drops per ounce of a spray bottle with water – but shake well before each use (oil and water separate!). Diffuse it on your patio.

Rosemary

Use This – <u>ROSEMARY</u> – For That

Use This for MEMORY & ALERTNESS

Use This for DEPRESSION & FATIGUE

Use This for NUMBNESS & PAIN

Use This as Your ASTRINGENT

Use This for ATTENTIVENESS, LIVELINESS & JOY

Use This to FIGHT COLDS, FLU & CONGESTION

Latin Name: Rosmarinus officinalis Leaves & twigs are Steam Distilled

MEMORY, ALERTNESS: Several recent clinical studies using Rosemary tested increase in attentiveness, alertness, liveliness, cognitive improvement and joyfulness. A number of studies have proven out these qualities, and in fact Rosemary is known through the ages as affecting memory – even Shakespeare mentioned this!

Diffuse often, inhale or use on your aromatherapy jewelry. Put 5-7 drops in an ounce of your favorite cream or oil.

DEPRESSION, FATIGUE, UPLIFT: Feeling depressed, fatigued, uninspired or just "blah"? Research shows Rosemary (along with a few other essential oils) can be nicely uplifting! Use it any way you wish, but diffusion is a smart way to go.

NUMB JOINTS, TIGHTNESS? Early Herbalists in Europe recommended Rosemary for this condition. You might want to blend 4-5 drops Rosemary with 2 drops Frankincense and 1 drop Turmeric into an ounce of cream and massage on those joints. Try drops of Rosemary in a warm soak for joints as well. Try a warm compress as well.

Related to this, some aromatherapists recommend using Rosemary during exercise class (apply a dilution on your skin or diffuse) as it helps prevent soreness or tightness that can occur.

COLDS & FLU? Add Rosemary to your list of essential oils to diffuse and kill airborne microbes. It is nice to change it up from day to day (Frankincense, Lemon, Eucalyptus, Lavender, Rosemary, etc.) and enjoy different aromas while purifying the air. Also, consider adding a drop to an aromatherapy necklace and breathe in as you need!

ASTRINGENT: Rosemary is also an astringent. Use it if you have oily skin or hair – put a few drops in your shampoo or cleansing toner. You might find that Tea Tree or Lemon work better, but experiment, especially if you like the scent and other qualities (including joyfulness it imparts!)

Ylang Ylang

Use This – <u>YLANG YLANG</u> – For That

Use for APHRODISIAC, EUPHORIA

Use This for INCREASED BLOOD FLOW

Use This for RAPID HEARTBEAT

Use This for INFLAMMATION

Use This for HELPING WITH PMS

Possible Use for EPILEPSY

Latin name: Canaga Odorata Production: Steam Distilled flowers

At the beginning of the 20th century, two French chemists and researchers discovered Ylang Ylang (most people pronounce this "lang lang") when conducting research on the Ile de Reunion. They discovered it was an effective treatment for all types of diseases including malaria, typhus and intestinal infections.

APHRODISIAC: Ylang Ylang is the most popular aphrodisiac among the essential oils in the West. Diffuse it in your bedroom, make a body oil or cream with 4-5 drops per ounce (it is strong.)

CIRCULATION AND BLOOD FLOW: Ylang Ylang helps generate circulation and better blood flow, good for libido but also for heart and body functions.

CALM FAST HEARTBEAT: The French researchers discovered its calming effect on the heart during times of distress (slowing a racing heart, helping to reduce stress.)

INFLAMMATION: The components include anti-inflammatory powers, helpful in a body massage or in a hot soak.

PMS: Ylang Ylang can help with the symptoms of PMS. Diffuse it, put some drops on your aromatherapy jewelry during difficult times, inhale as needed. Certainly using drops (6) in an ounce of cream could help, massage on your body!

EPILEPSY: Ylang Ylang is being studied as a potentially effective essential oil for epilepsy, as shown in clinical trials performed by Dr. Betts of England. However, if you suffer from epilepsy, please consult with your doctor on this.

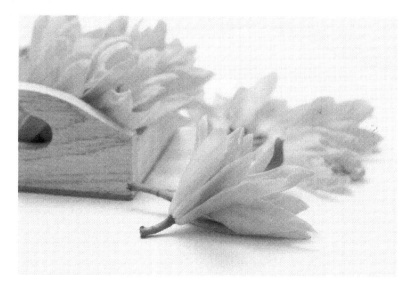

Eucalyptus

Use This – <u>EUCALYPTUS</u> – For That

Use This For SINUSES & CONGESTION

Use This For COLDS & FLU

Use This for a Superior BACTERICIDE & ANTISEPTIC

Use This For INVIGORATION, TO ENERGIZE, TO SOOTHE FATIGUE

Use This For HELPING FOCUS & CONCENTRATION

Latin name: Eucalyptus Globulus Steam Distillation (leaves)

Eucalyptus is one of the essential oils everyone should have – and many people are familiar with. It's powerful, fresh and medicinal.

SINUS, COUGHS & CONGESTION: Eucalyptus is superior for respiratory and sinus support, for its antibacterial and antifungal powers, and for wellness support.

Diffuse Eucalyptus, inhale it or do a steam tent several times daily (7-8 drops) if you feel a cold coming on.

If you have ongoing sinus problems, start using Eucalyptus inhalations every few hours during the day; diffuse at night, and/or make a cream with 7 drops to an ounce. Put a drop on your

34

temples and under your nostrils at night, and include your chest if you have congestion or respiratory issues. For coughs, blend Eucalyptus (4 drops) and Cedarwood (3 drops) and diffuse.

If you have sick people around you, diffuse it for protection!

I love to put some drops in the corner of the shower floor (where you will NOT step or slip on it), and let it rise with the steam and help congestion – or just for the invigoration!

BACTERICIDE. Study after study of Eucalyptus shows us its strong antibacterial powers. To cite just one study, researchers at Australia's Royal Brisbane & Women's Hospital tested Eucalyptus (also Tea Tree and Lemongrass) against antibiotic-resistant superbugs. They also tested common antiseptics used at hospitals (rubbing alcohol) at the same time. The Essential Oils had large zones of inhibition of the superbugs – far superior results than the rubbing alcohol.

Use some drops in the washer or dryer to freshen and cleanse towels and sheets – after someone has been sick in the home, or if you had houseguests. Diffuse it. Use it on some aromatherapy jewelry.

FATIGUED, TIRED, SORE, HAVE MELANCHOLY?
Eucalyptus is great to help revive you. It is simply invigorating and makes you feel good. Inhale or diffuse - plus if you have muscular tiredness, you can put 5-6 drops in your favorite oil or cream and massage to set yourself right.

FOCUS & CONCENTRATION: Eucalyptus is a good choice to diffuse if you want to concentrate or focus on something.

Star Anise

Use This – <u>STAR ANISE</u> – For That

Use This For VIRAL INFECTIONS

Use This For FLU, COUGH, COLDS

Use This For BACTERIAL STRAINS

Use This For YEAST INFECTIONS

Use This For INDIGESTION, GAS

Use This for LIBIDO

Use This for RHEUMATISM & LOWER BACK PAIN

Use This for IMMUNE SUPPORT

Latin Name: Illicium Verum Steam Distilled

Star Anise is less known in the U.S., but is very well known and used in Asia.

ANTI-VIRAL THANKS TO SHIKIMIC ACID: Star Anise is the primary source of shikimic acid in the world, a plant-based compound that is the precursor to oseltamivir, an antiviral medication that is marketed as Tamiflu, according to an article in a 2011 issue of "Alternative Medicine Studies." Although shikimic acid also occurs naturally in ginkgo and sweetgum fruit, Star Anise has far greater concentrations. In fact, <u>without Star Anise, there is</u>

36

no Tamiflu.

Diffuse it, inhale it. Make a body cream (6-8 drops per ounce) and massage on your check, neck, and body.

FLU, COLDS, COUGHS, STRONG ANTIBACTERIAL: In addition to being an anti-viral, Star Anise is also exceptional for treating coughs due to asthma and bronchitis because it has expectorant properties. It has been shown to be effective against 67 drug resistant bacterial strains (Journal of Medicinal Food.)

Diffuse it, inhale it, use it when those around you are sick, or as a preventive. It has a licorice-type scent and many kids may like it when they are sick. Note that you can add a drop of Cedarwood to Star Anise for coughing issues.

YEAST INFECTIONS: Star Anise is potent against yeast, and well tested in the East. Massage your body with 10 drops of Star Anise to an ounce of your favorite oil or cream. Diffuse it, and put some in your bath soak.

INDIGESTION, GAS: While we tend to think of Peppermint in the West for this; the East uses Star Anise for problems such as bloating, abdominal cramps, gas, indigestion and constipation and also activates the metabolic enzymes. You can put 7 drops in a cream or oil and massage on your abdomen, and also inhale deeply. It blends well with Peppermint, so you can do 4-5 drops Star Anise to 3 drops Peppermint!

RHEUMATISM: Star Anise has been found to be beneficial in patients with rheumatism and also with lower back pain. Regular massage with the oil (6-7 drops per ounce) could help with the pain and inflammation.

LIBIDO: Star Anise is sometimes used to help increase libido in the East.

IMMUNE SUPPORT: Italian researchers tested shikimic acid alone and in combination with quercetin, an antioxidant-rich plant-based nutrient, to see if they could bolster immune function to help fight off flu or other viral infections. The two combined, even at low doses, helped ramp up immune function to better resist viral infection. Researchers published their findings in the April 2008 issue of "Journal of Medical Virology." In addition, the qualities of Star Anise can help bolster the overall immune system.

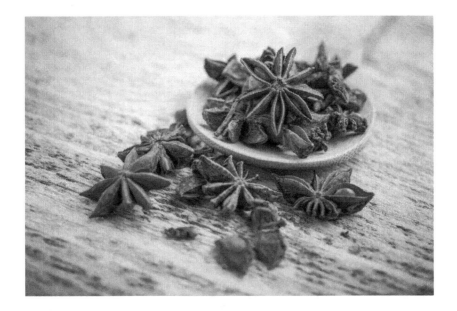

Clary Sage

Use This – <u>CLARY SAGE</u> – For That

Use This For FEMALE HORMONAL SUPPORT

Use This For An APHRODISIAC

Use This For INFLAMMATION

Use This for a Strong ANTI-STAPHYLOCCAL

Use This for HEADACHES

Use This For FIGHTING ADDICTION

Use This For Better CIRCULATION

Use This for CARDIO-PROTECTIVE & CHOLESTEROL

Use This for ASTHMA & COUGHING OR SPASMS

Use This For INDIGESTION

Use This (With Lavender) for INSOMNIA and ANXIETY

Use This For RELAXING THE MIND & MEDITATION

May Help Fight LEUKEMIA

Latin name: Salvia Sclarea Steam Distilled (leaves and/ or flowers)

CAUTIONS: Clary Sage is widely reported to increase the narcotic

39

effects of alcohol and should therefore be avoided if drinking or driving. In addition, due to its estrogenic nature, Clary Sage could have a negative impact on people who need to regulate their estrogen levels. Seek the advice of your healthcare advisor before using, if you are on estrogen or hormonal treatments.

Clary Sage is actually considered to be the top essential oil for female hormone support. It can help with cramps, hot flashes and hormonal imbalances (and is recommended for this in France.)

CRAMPS, MENSTRUAL ISSUES, HORMONAL IMBALANCE? Many health issues today, even things like infertility, polycystic ovary syndrome and estrogen-based cancers, are caused from <u>excess estrogen</u> in the body — in part because of our consumption of high-estrogen foods. Because Clary Sage helps balance out those estrogen levels, it could help. Inhale or diffuse as needed.

<u>Create a massage oil</u> by diluting 5-7 drops of Clary Sage oil with 5 drops of a carrier oil (like jojoba or coconut oil) and apply it to needed areas. If you have a bad case of cramps, also inhale or diffuse.

APHRODISIAC: Clary Sage is a substance or stimulus that boosts libido and feelings of sexual desire. It is very effective in treating frigidity, psychological problems resulting in loss of libido, and even impotency. Note that Ylang Ylang and Neroli are two other oils recommended as aphrodisiacs.

INFLAMMATION, MUSCULAR or JOINT PAIN: Add 7 drops of Clary Sage oil to warm bath water – or on your bath salts! You could also use it in a warm compress. Can be blended with Frankincense as well to reduce inflammation.

STRONG ANTI-STAPHYLOCCAL and ANTI-BACTERIAL: A 2015 medical study showed Clary Sage Essential Oil may be effectively applied to treat wounds and skin infections due to its antimicrobial properties. It indicated a strong anti-staphylococcal activity against clinical strains isolated from wound infections — the oil was active against strains, including Staphylococcus aureus, S. epidermidis and S. xylosus.

It's also a good anti-bacterial (like most essential oils). Diffuse to purify the air, or if sick ones are in the home, or inhale while travelling. For wounds, use in a compress, or put drops in a gel, jojoba or carrier to treat a wound.

HEADACHES & MIGRAINES: Thanks to its circulation aid and properties to relax, Clary Sage could help reduce headaches and migraines. Use on a compress (7 drops in water, wring out the cloth and put on forehead) and/or inhale.

FIGHT ADDICTION: Clary Sage Essential Oil has been used to battle addiction (particularly drugs) and can stimulate a change in mentality towards a positive way of approaching life.

INCREASE CIRCULATION. Clary Sage opens the blood vessels and allows for increased blood circulation; it also naturally lowers blood pressure by relaxing the brain and arteries. This boosts the performance of the metabolic system by increasing the amount of oxygen that gets into the muscles and supporting organ function.

CARDIO-PROTECTIVE & REDUCE CHOLESTEROL: Cholesterol is a naturally occurring substance made by the liver and required by the body for the proper function of cells, nerves and hormones. Cholesterol travels in the lipids (fatty acids) of the bloodstream, which is also called plaque, and can build up in the walls of the arteries, decreasing blood flow. <u>The antioxidant and anti-inflammatory properties of Clary Sage oil are cardio-protective and help lower cholesterol naturally</u>. Clary Sage also decreases emotional stress and improves circulation, which can help in reducing cholesterol and supporting the cardiovascular system.

ASTHMA, COUGH, SPASMS: Clary Sage is used for respiratory issues, such as asthma. The oil is often used in asthma blends, as it relieves spasms in the chest and helps ease anxiety that can come with asthma. It also helps circulation and inflammation. Of course, we caution any asthmatic when using essential oils, and you may wish to check with your doctor or aromatherapist first.

INDIGESTION: We tend to think of Peppermint first for indigestion, but Clary Sage can help as well. Clary Sage <u>boosts the secretion of gastric juices </u>and bile, which speeds up and eases the digestive process. By relieving symptoms of indigestion, it minimizes cramping, bloating and abdominal discomfort. It can also prevents stomach disorders and helps the body to absorb the much-needed vitamins and minerals that are consumed throughout the day. It regulates bowel movements and relieves constipation. Use 10 drops in a cream or oil and massage on your tummy and abdomen before and after eating + inhale.

INSOMNIA & ANXIETY. Clary Sage is a natural sedative and helps to calm for good sleep. Diffuse or apply, excellent to use with Lavender. <u>Especially good if your cause of insomnia is stress or hormonal change-related.</u> In addition, Clary Sage can bring down cortisol levels (like Rosemary does), and this can help calm anxiety or stress.

RELAX THE MIND, MEDITATION: For meditation or to enhance healing prayer, mix 6 drops of Clary Sage oil with 2 drops of Frankincense. Use in a diffuser or make a blend in a cream or oil and use on the body before meditation.

If you are stressed or your mind is going in a thousand directions, diffuser Clary Sage or Clary Sage + Frankincense.

A NOTE ON LEUKEMIA: The Department of Immunology, Hellenic Anticancer Institute in Athens, Greece, examined the role that sclareol, a chemical compound found in Clary Sage, plays in fighting leukemia. The results showed that sclareol is able to kill cell lines through the process of apoptosis. Apoptosis is the process of programmed cell death; research involving the role of apoptosis has increased substantially since the early 1990s. An insufficient amount of apoptosis results in uncontrolled cell proliferation, such as cancer.

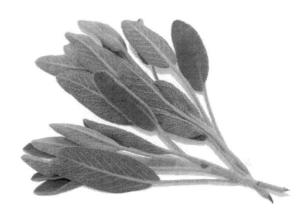

Bergamot

USE THIS – <u>BERGAMOT</u> – FOR THAT

Use This For **URINARY TRACT INFECTIONS**

Use This For **HEADACHES**

Use This for **COUGHS & SPASMS**

Use This For **GAS, CRAMPS & DIGESTIVE STIMULATION**

Use This For **RESTLESS LEG SYNDROME**

Use This For **SORE MUSCLES**

Use This To **CLEANSE FRUITS & VEGGIES**

Use This If **FEELING BLUE OR STRESSED FOR UPLIFT**

Latin Name: Citrus Bergamia. Cold Pressed Peels

Bergamot is a lovely, lesser-known citric essential oil which is sweeter and softer than most other citrus. Almost everyone who discovers it falls in love!

URINARY TRACT INFECTION & ANTI-MICROBIAL:
The Journal of Applied Microbiology published that Bergamot produced positive results against Enterococcus faecium & Enterococcus faecalis bacteria, potent antibiotic-resistant microbes. These enterococcal species are a common source of a variety of infections, including urinary tract infections (UTI), bacteremia,

endocarditis, and meningitis.

Add 10-12 drops of Bergamot to your sitz bath or hip bath to help prevent the spread of bacterial infections from the urethra into the bladder. It has shown great effectiveness against the specific bacteria that causes these infections.

HEADACHES: Use a cold compress with 6 drops of Bergamot (or blend 4 Bergamot and 2 Lavender) for relief. Swish your cloth or washcloth in a bowl of water with the drops, wring it out and put on your forehead. Freshen as needed. Use can also diffuse it.

ANTI-SPASMODIC, COUGHS: Bergamot is an anti-spasmodic and can help calm coughs. Diffuse it, do a steam tent; inhale it directly from the bottle.

RESTLESS LEG SYNDROME: Bergamot has been shown to help! Put Bergamot in a carrier oil and massage your legs. A 3% dilution is good, which means 15 drops in one ounce of carrier. Use as often as needed. If using at night, you might want to use a cream or gel instead of oil.

DIGESTIVE CRAMPS, GAS, ISSUES: Bergamot is also known to help with abdominal cramps and digestive discomfort such as excess gas. Make a blend with 10 drops in a carrier and massage on your tummy. Diffuse as well.

In a study published in the Journal of Antimicrobial Chemotherapy, Italian researchers have proven Bergamot Essential Oil's amazing antifungal properties when used as a topical remedy for infections brought by candida fungus strains, which can be behind some digestive issues.

CLEANSE FRUITS & VEGGIES: Similar to our suggestion with Lemon Essential Oil, use Bergamot to cleanse against pesticides, toxins and things like salmonella! Add 3-4 drops of

Bergamot to half a gallon of water and cleanse – then rinse!

FEELING BLUE OR STRESSED? It's an anti-depressant and helps bring you out of the doldrums or grief. It is a happy scent that is bright and is great for emotional support – I diffuse it once in a while and always enjoy the experience.

Lovely Recipe for an Anti-Depressant: Blend 3 drops Bergamot with 2 drop Lavender and 1 drop Ylang Ylang. Diffuse!

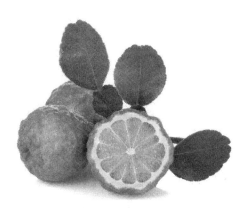

Rose Geranium

USE THIS – <u>ROSE GERANIUM</u> – FOR THAT

Use This For GRIEF & SADNESS

Use This For LYMPHATIC SUPPORT

Use This For FACIAL SKIN CARE

Use This For INFLAMMATION or SWELLING

Use This For A BLEEDING CUT & WOUND HEALING

Use This For SCARS & STRETCH MARKS

Latin Name: Pelargonium graveolans Leaves & Stems Steam Distilled

GRIEF, DEPRESSION: Rose Geranium is specifically known to help with grief and sadness. Diffuse or inhale periodically during such a period. It is very balancing yet uplifting. If you are going through a sad period, following a death, for instance, use in the diffuser but make a topical and apply to your wrists & neck or pulse points. Mix 10 drops in an ounce of carrier. Put some drops on your aromatherapy jewelry.

LYMPHATIC SUPPORT: Rose Geranium has a gentle stimulating effect on the lymphatic system – it can help with fluid retention and circulation as well as regulating effects. Excellent to use after <u>Skin Brushing</u> (which also supports the lymphatic system.)

FACIAL SKIN CARE: Add 6-7 drops per ounce of your face cream or oil. I typically use Frankincense in my night cream, but I

48

do have a small jar with Rose Geranium that I love to use in the morning and on weekends. It helps with inflammation, promotes circulation (great for skin tone), also relieves dryness and works on wrinkles.

BLEEDING CUT, WOUND HEALING, ANTISEPTIC: Rose Geranium could be used neat after a patch test. Though I typically use Lavender if I cut myself, I use Rose Geranium if the cut is bleeding more than usual – Rose Geranium speeds up clotting. It is a nice antibacterial to help cleanse the wound and help it heal, too.

INFLAMMATION OR SWELLING: We know that Frankincense is making inroads for sufferers of Arthritis and Rheumatoid Arthritis. Because Rose Geranium helps with inflammation, you can add several drops to your organic cream or oil in addition to Frankincense, to help reduce inflammation. Nice in a hand cream!

Rose Geranium can be used in a nice cool foot soak to help reduce the inflammation - or add 7 drops to your body cream or oil and massage on your feet, ankles and calves.

SCARS & STRETCH MARKS: Rose Geranium is a powerful cicatrisant (that is, helps the fading of scars, marks and issues on the skin). It increases blood circulation just below the skin (which helps with healing and skin tone). Put 10-12 drops in 1 ounce of a carrier and apply 3 times daily. We find Baobab Oil the best for this purpose since Baobab is also known as a scar reducer. Other oils like Jojoba would be perfectly fine, too.

Turmeric

Use This – <u>TURMERIC</u> – For That

Use This For INFLAMMATION, ARTHRITIS

Use This For ACHY OR SWOLLEN FEET & ANKLE

Use This For ANTI-FUNGAL POWER

Use This For IBS

Use This For RECOVERY FROM A VIRAL INFECTION

Use This For SLUGGISH LIVER / SLUGGISH DIGESTION

Use This For WARMING, GROUNDING SPIRIT

_____

Latin Name: Curcuma longa Steam or CO2 Distillation of the root

ARTHRITIS, INFLAMMATION: Put 10-11 drops of
Turmeric in an organic cream, and massage on the affected area.
Include 4 drops of frankincense if desired.

Turmeric extract <u>worked as well as a non-steroidal anti-
inflammatory drug for treatment of osteoarthritis</u> of the knee in a
study published in the August 2009 issue of the Journal of
Alternative and Complementary Medicine.

Do a patch test, and you may be able to use it "neat" on swollen
fingers from time to time when pain flares up.

If you suffer from arthritis or rheumatoid arthritis, diffuse Turmeric
from time to time. It is not typically diffused as the scent is rooty
and medicinal, yet give it a go if you are suffering.

FOOT BATH. Put drops of Turmeric into your bath or foot bath
and take a soak! Great if you are achy or inflamed. Include 10
drops of Turmeric, and you can add 4 drops Frankincense and/or 4
drops Rose Geranium.

ANTI-FUNGAL. Though we tend to use Tea Tree to attack
fungus, Turmeric has been shown to have excellent powers in this
area and is used in the East, especially India, for this purpose.

IBS? Turmeric is an essential oil that could help (like Peppermint).
Blend 6-10 drops it into an ounce of oil or cream and massage on
your belly. Curcumin (the active ingredient in Turmeric) suppresses
micro-inflammation in the GI tract associated with inflammatory
bowel disease

51

RECOVERY FROM A VIRAL INFECTION? Turmeric has been shown to help in the recovery from a viral infection. Use it in a massage (6-10 drops per ounce), diffuse and/or use it in a soak.

SLUGGISH LIVER/SLUGGISH DIGESTION: Turmeric could help with liver congestion, cleansing and sluggish digestion in moderation and in short bouts – use it in an oil or cream and massage on your mid-section at a higher dilution that normal (say 12-15 drops) except if you are on blood thinners or suffer from a bile disease.

WARMING, GROUNDING, SOOTHING: Turmeric is a warming essential oil, like its cousin Ginger. It can help the spirit feel grounded, warm and cozy. It can also focus scattered energy. Finally, it can soothe the spirit, calm anger and relax.

Chapter 3
SPECIFIC WELLNESS ISSUES

This chapter is arranged by specific issue, such as headaches, stress or coughs.

At the beginning of the page for each condition, you will find the list of various essential oils used in the section. Then you will see various suggestions or recipes to try for the problem! I also note a few of my personal favorites as well.

Headaches form the longest section, as there are so many different types, it is such a common problem, and there are many tested essential oils for the problem.

COMPRESS: I sometimes suggest a cold or warm compress. The most typical method here is to have water in a small bowl (warm or cold), put in the suggested drops, swish your washcloth or compress in it; wring it out then apply.

TIP: You will note that many (if not all) essential oils are anti-bacterial in varying degrees, and can be used for similar conditions. I think it is smart to trade out or alternate different essential oils every so often, especially if dealing with a chronic situation (like chronic cough) or to purify the air of microbes during flu season. Expert Robert Tisserand alludes to this, saying it would be a smart practice to avoid the body getting too used to one essential oil or the other.

HEADACHES

ESSENTIAL OILS IN THIS SECTION: EUCALYPTUS, LAVENDER, PEPPERMINT, CLARY SAGE, ROSEMARY, PEPPERMINT, BERGAMOT, BASIL, MAY CHANG, LEMON, CARDAMON, ROMAN CHAMOMILE, TURMERIC, CAJUPUT, GINGER, FRANKINCENSE, YLANG YLANG, ROSE GERANIUM, TEA TREE, CLOVE, LEMONGRASS, GRAPEFRUIT, PETIT GRAIN, HELICHRYSUM

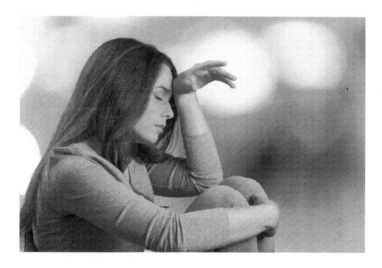

Did you know that there are 150 different types of headaches?

Different types of headaches are typically handled in different ways.

We won't list all of the types, but here are the most common:

A **tension headache** is a most common form of general headache caused by stress and tension.

Sinus headaches, caused by inflammation of the sinus cavity (sometimes this occurs with a runny nose, cold, or even a specific allergy which produces too much mucus).

Migraines, often described as powerful and pounding which can last for hours or even days and might be triggered by something or recur. During a migraine, an upset stomach might occur, and even sensitivity to sound and light.

Cluster headaches typically give a piercing or harsh pain in the head, may be behind the eye, and may be throbbing. The face may flush and eyes water. (They are called cluster because they often repeat or come back frequently in a certain amount of days.) Alcohol and tobacco are two culprits, and apparently men get cluster headaches more than women, according to the National Headache Foundation. http://www.headaches.org/2008/12/11/the-complete-headache-chart/

Fever headaches are brought on during fever when blood vessels are swollen in the head.

Mixed Headache Syndrome is typically a migraine mixed with a tension headache.

Allergy headaches typically happen during certain times of the year during seasonal periods.

Hormone headaches typically occur during pregnancy, periods or menopause when hormones levels are changing.

Arthritis headaches typically occur in the back of the neck or head, caused by inflammation of the bones and restriction of blood flow.

Hangover headaches are caused due to dilation of and irritation of blood vessels from alcohol.

Hunger headaches can occur when blood sugar drops, from muscle tension, skipping a meal, oversleeping or poor diet.

Hypertension headaches most often occur in the morning, and can be suffered by those with high blood pressure

TMJ (temporomandibular) headaches could occur in those suffering with TMJ, with muscle contraction of the jaw, poor alignment or related.

General Exertion headaches may occur after physical exertion, strenuous exercise, or even passive exertion like coughing.

Depression headaches are most commonly related to tension or anxiety headaches, brought on my depression, negative feelings or anxiety – all perhaps repressed or hidden.

Chronic daily headaches refers to a headache that occurs more than 15 days per month.

Different things can trigger headaches in different people. If you suffer often, keep a diary and try to pinpoint what triggers your headache (a certain food or drink, for instance, or a certain type of pollen or environment.) This can help you try to avoid or prevent, and gives you information to share with your doctor if you need to.

If you have an ongoing headache, or something that progressively becomes worse, seek out a doctor who may want to test.

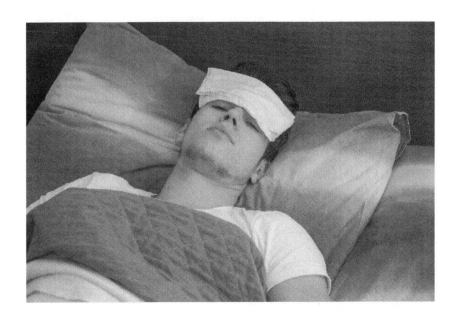

SOME ESSENTIAL OILS TO TRY FOR YOUR HEADACHE

MY PERSONAL FAVORITES: I rarely get headaches, but if I do it tends to be sinus-related. I adore using Eucalyptus to take care of it.

Headache Due to Sinus Problems: If you suffer from ongoing sinus problems or colds, start addressing it with EUCALYPTUS inhalations every few hours. At night, you can diffuse EUCALYPTUS or make up a cream or oil (7 drops per ounce) and apply to chest and temples before bed. It can be a little stimulating but will also help with respiration and kill bacteria that may be causing the sinus infections.

Sinus Headache II: CAJUPUT essential oil could help. Diffuse it, or do a steam tent several times daily, or a warm bath with 7 drops.

General Headache/Tension: You can try a cold compress with 5 drops of PEPPERMINT. You could also add 3 drops of LAVENDER to the water if desired. Put the drops of essential oil in a cool water bowl, swish your washcloth or compress in the water with the essential oils; wring it out and apply to your forehead. Keep out of your eyes.

General Headache: Use a cold compress with 4-5 drops of BERGAMOT (or blend BERGAMOT and 2 drops of LAVENDER) for relief. It will help reduce inflammation and soothe the spirit.

General Headache/Tension Headache: Traditional Chinese medicine uses MAY CHANG (Litsea Cubeba) to treat tension conditions. Do a cold compress with 5-6 drops of MAY CHANG.

Tension Headache Blend (*courtesy Aromahead Institute*):

3 drops Lavender   6 drops Frankincense
2 drops Rosemary   1 drop Eucalyptus (globulus)
1 drop Helichrysum

Blend in 1 oz. of cream or oil. Rub on the back of your neck and temples as soon as tension begins.

Migraine: Try CLARY SAGE, LEMON, LAVENDER, MAJORAM, PEPPERMINT OR ROMAN CHAMOMILE. A cold compress in a dark, quiet room may help and you can also diffuse your favorite essential oils from the list. Choose one that you like and favor when you don't have your headache, something you resonate with. Use 6 drops for your compress.

Note About the Two Most Suggested Essential Oils for Migraines: Thanks to the circulation aid, and properties to relax, CLARY SAGE is often recommended for migraines. LEMON also improves circulation and is "cleansing". Diffuse either, use in a bath, use on a compress.

Depression Headache: Try YLANG YLANG, CLARY SAGE, the CITRUSES, ROSE GERANIUM, ROSEMARY or FRANKINCENSE. These are essential oils that help with depression, and bring uplift. Diffuse, inhale, do a cool compress with 5-6 drops in water; or mix 5-6 drops in an ounce of your carrier and apply to temples, forehead, back of neck and wrists.

Various Headaches: BASIL is an essential oil that can help reduce or stop a headache. Inhale it, and then use one of the two applications here: 1) do a cool compress with several drops of BASIL and relax in a darkened room. 2) For a stress or tension headache, put several 4-5 drops of BASIL (you can also include 1 drop of FRANKINCENSE or ROSEMARY) into an ounce of cream or oil, and massage it on your neck, temples and forehead lightly.

General Headache: ROMAN or GERMAN CHAMOMILE may help, as well as ROSEWOOD or LEMONGRASS

Fever Headaches: Do a cold compress of LEMONGRASS, or LEMON or PALMAROSA (used in India for fevers & inflammation) or EUCALYPTUS (once called "fever oil") or PEPPERMINT (except for babies or young children – peppermint is too strong for them.) Drink lots of water to hydrate, use a cold pack or even ice bath with one of the essential oils above, if necessary.

Exhaustion Headache: If nerves are jangled, you are tired or overworked and developed a headache, try a diffusion and/or cold compress of LAVENDER, NEROLI, or CLARY SAGE. Use 5 drops of your chosen oil.

Hunger Headache: Give GRAPEFRUIT, PEPPERMINT, CINNAMON, CLOVE or SWEET ORANGE a try! Simply inhale deeply three times in each nostril. You can repeat every 30-45 minutes or as needed.

Hangover Headache: Soak in a bath with GRAPEFRUIT and/or ROSEMARY. You could also do a cold compress with the same essential oils (5-7 drops.)

Hypertension Headache: Try LAVENDER, YLANG YLANG, CLARY SAGE and/or FRANKINCENSE. These are all calming essential oils that can help reduce oxidative stress plus they are physically relaxing.

Allergy Headache: You may want to change air conditioning filters and even drip EUCALYPTUS, LEMON or TEA TEA on them (or diffuse in the air duct) to kill off potential allergens in your home. Inhale or diffuse EUCALYPTUS or CLOVE (or blend them equally, 4 drops each in your diffuser.) Use often during allergy season or when suffering.

Allergy Headache II: Try diffusing or inhaling ROSE GERANIUM and TEA TREE essential oils; or just PEPPERMINT. These have all helped allergy headaches.

Allergy Headache III: Try a pre-blend like our Zen Allergy & Immune Response with LAVENDER, LIME, EUCALYPUS, ROSEMARY, GINGER, PEPPERMINT & CARDAMOM. It's a pre-emptive blend during allergy season that could help with a headache as well. Put drops under your nostrils, on your pulse points. Inhale.

TMJ Headache: Give LAVENDER a go, or try a blend already mixed like the Zen DeStress Essential Oil Blend with LAVENDER to help reduce the tension and stress on the jaw line. Massage on your jaw area, and you can also diffuse.

Arthritis Headache: Try TURMERIC or GINGER topically (6 drops in an ounce of cream, massage on); or use LAVENDER and/or FRANKINCENSE in a compress or diffusion (5-6 drops).

Hormonal Headache: Try CLARY SAGE for any hormonal type headache. Inhale or diffuse!

General Exertion Headaches: Try FRANKINCENSE or ROSEMARY for this. Diffuse, or apply a body lotion with 5-7 drops in an ounce after exercise or exertion. (You could add 1 drop of LAVENDER if desired.)

Chronic Headaches or Recurring Headaches: Put together your own balm or cream to use proactively or when a headache starts to develop. Blend 2 drops of PEPPERMINT, 5 drops of LAVENDER and 4 drops of EUCALYPTUS in 1 ½ ounces of cream or gel. Or try 4 drops of PETITGRAIN and 6 drops LAVENDER in 1 ½ ounces of cream or gel.

COLDS, FLU & CONGESTION

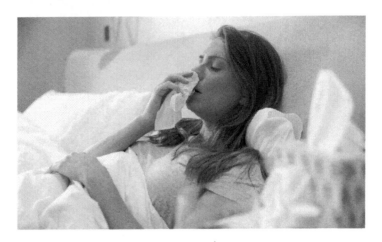

ESSENTIAL OILS IN THIS SECTION: EUCALYPTUS, CINNAMON, CLOVE, SIBERIAN PINE NEEDLE, LEMONGRASS, STAR ANISE, OREGANO, BERGAMOT, ROSEMARY, CEDARWOOD, LAVENDER, LEMON, TEA TREE

MY PERSONAL FAVORITES: I rarely get a cold or flu anymore, but if I travel or feel one coming on, my personal favorite is a mix of EUCALYPUS and CLOVE. I also like SIBERIAN PINE NEEDLE, as it has good powers for respiratory problems and makes me feel like I am in a forest at Christmas!

If you feel a cold coming on, immediately use EUCALYPTUS in a steam blend (a steam tent or breath in from your diffuser) for a few days, two to four times a day (or more). You can also breathe in deeply directly from your bottle or an inhaler often. It's also preventative for cold or flu. And if you have sick people around you, diffuse for protection!

If you suffer from ongoing sinusitis, as mentioned in the previous section under sinus headaches, address it with EUCALYPTUS inhalations. At night, you can diffuse it or, make a cream or oil (4 drops in 2 ounces) and apply to chest and temples before bed. It can be a little stimulating but will also help with respiration and killing bacteria that may be causing the sinus infections.

Researchers at Cornell University found that LAVENDER oil can eradicate certain antibiotic-resistant bacteria, including more than one strain of pathogenic Staphylococcus and **pathogenic Streptococcus (often involved in coughs and colds**). Diffuse it! Also excellent at night for better sleep when you may have a cold.

Cold or Flu with Coughing? CEDARWOOD is superior for treating coughs suffered along with a cold or flu, shown after extensive studies in France. Inhale, diffuse; do a steam tent 3 times daily; put 7-10 drops in a cream and use on your throat, upper chest, and sinus areas.

Flu with some coughing that may be due to mold, fungal issues or allergies? Inhale TEA TREE which can excel in addressing (especially fungus, mold, allergies, but also bacteria or viruses.) In addition, several medical studies show that TEA TREE can help treat flu and actually has an **inhibitory effect on H1N1 flu**. Diffuse, and/or mix drops in a carrier oil and massage on your chest and throat.

Flu in the House? Use ROSEMARY essential oil to diffuse and kill airborne microbes. It is nice to change it up from day to day when there are sick ones in the house, and to alternate with EUCALYPTUS, OREGANO, CLOVE & LAVENDER. Enjoy different aromas while purifying the air and staying well, or helping your family get better.

Anti-Viral: STAR ANISE is the primary source of shikimic acid, a plant-based compound that is the precursor to oseltamivir, an antiviral medication that is marketed as Tamiflu. Although shikimic acid also occurs naturally in ginkgo and sweetgum fruit, STAR ANISE has far greater concentrations. <u>As mentioned in chapter 2, without it, there is no Tamiflu</u>. Diffuse it, inhale it often, put 5-6 drops in a cream or oil and apply to neck, temples & chest.

Protect Against Infections or Reduce Effects of Flu:
CINNAMON supports the body against infections like the flu and colds. If you do get a flu, then use CINNAMON to help <u>reduce the effects</u>. Use it in a warm bath daily, or compresses and definitely diffuse it!

COUGHS, BRONCHIAL ISSUES

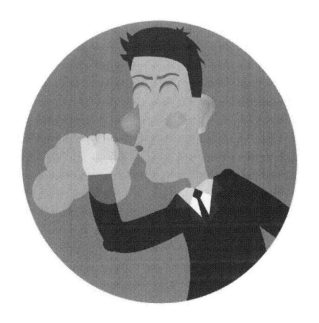

ESSENTIAL OILS IN THIS SECTION: CEDARWOOD, EUCALYPTUS, MYRRH, HELICHRYSUM, BERGAMOT, SIBERIAN PINE NEEDLE, MAY CHANG, TEA TREE, BASIL, CLOVE, STAR ANISE, LEMON, FRANKINCENSE

PERSONAL FAVORITES: I do suffer from coughs from time to time due to sensitivity to salt and dry throat. My personal favorites are CEDARWOOD, MYRRH & HELICHRYSUM to help.

Ongoing Respiratory Issues? You could benefit from using FRANKINCENSE on a regular basis in different formats: put some in your body cream, in your aromatherapy jewelry, diffuse, use in a bath or foot soak. It can also help to clear phlegm – use 5-7 drops in your cream or oil and massage on the throat, chest and even temples; do a tent steam!

A Cough Recipe – GARGLE: blend 2 drop of TEA TREE with 2 drop of EUCALYPTUS and 1 drop of LEMON in a teaspoon of honey, then dilute in a <u>cup of very warm water and gargle</u>!

Chronic Bronchitis, Coughing or Agitation: French physicians reported good results with CEDARWOOD use in cases of chronic bronchitis. Diffuse it and/or inhale from the bottle or personal inhaler often if suffering. Put 7-10 drops in an ounce of body cream, gel or oil and massage on your chest, throat, back of neck and wrists.

Bronchitis, Cough Due to Bacterial Infection or Asthma: STAR ANISE, a strong anti-viral, is also quite effective treating cough due to asthma and bronchitis due to its expectorant property. Is has been shown to be effective against 67 drug resistant bacterial strains (Journal of Medicinal Food.)

Mucus Cough? Inhale & diffuse 2-3 drops HELICHRYSUM and 4 drops MYRRH.

Pleasant Anti-Spasmodic. HELICYRYSUM is a wonderful essential oil. It is anti-spasmodic, brings warmth to the respiratory system and smells great. Diffuse, use 5 drops in a steam tent, or make a massage oil with 6-10 drops per ounce of carrier & massage on your neck & chest.

Researchers at Cornell University found that LAVENDER oil can eradicate certain antibiotic-resistant bacteria, including more than one strain of pathogenic Staphylococcus and pathogenic Streptococcus (often involved in coughs and colds).

Respiratory Issues with Frequent Coughing? BERGAMOT is an anti-spasmodic and can help calm coughs; SIBERIAN PINE NEEDLE helps coughing as does CEDARWOOD. Diffuse or inhale any of these, or alternate them out! Use about 6-7 drops in your diffuser.

Reduce Irritability While Fighting Cough & Cold: MAY CHANG (Litsea Cubeba) is great against cold and coughs! It is nicely uplifting and helps emotional stability and reduces irritability.

Respiratory Illnesses. If you have chronic respiratory issues, or a combination of cold, flu, sinus infection and coughing due to a respiratory problem, try BASIL. It helps ease coughing and spasms, it helps attack bacteria, it helps relieve sinuses and it's an expectorant.

Bronchitis. SIBERIAN PINE NEEDLE is helpful! Diffuse it, inhale it, put a little in a cream or oil and dot on your temples or use a compress. Include a drop of EUCALYPTUS or CLOVE if you wish.

Respiratory issues with frequent coughing? BERGAMOT is an anti-spasmodic and can help calm coughs; SIBERIAN PINE

NEEDLE helps coughing as does CEDARWOOD. Diffuse or inhale any of these, or alternate them out! Use about 6-7 drops in your diffuser.

SORE THROAT

ESSENTIAL OILS IN THIS SECTION: EUCALYPTUS, MYRRH, LAVENDER, ROSE GERANIUM, TEA TREE, THYME, CLOVE, CLARY SAGE, LEMON, CEDARWOOD

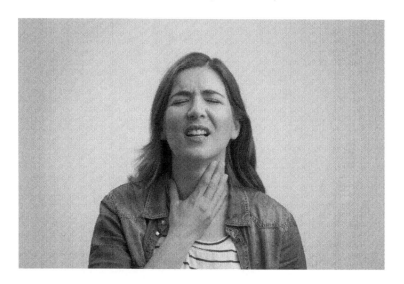

PERSONAL FAVORITES: My go-to is EUCALYPTUS, MYRRH or FRANKINCENSE.

SORE THROAT: A sore throat is often the first sign of a cold, flu or virus. I like to do a massage blend for the throat as follows: 10 drops EUCALYPTUS, 4 drops CEDARWOOD, 2 drops PINE NEEDLE, 2 drops ROSE GERANIUM in an ounce of a cream. Massage over throat, cover with a scarf. Repeat every few hours.

You can also keep it simple and just do a mix of EUCALYPTUS or just CEDARWOOD and massage on your throat.

STEAM TENT I: An immediate steam tent can help to soothe and kill bacteria. Do an infusion of EUCALYPTUS and CLOVE, 3-4 drops each.

STEAM TENT II: Do a steam tent of ROSE GERANIUM, CLARY SAGE and THYME 2-3 drops each.

STEAM TENT III: If you suspect fungi or mold may be part of the sore throat, do a steam tent with 4 drops TEA TREE and 2 drops ROSE GERANIUM.

GARGLE I: Gargling immediately can help. Put 1 drop of LEMON ESSENTIAL OIL and 1 drop of CLOVE OR MYRRH into 2 teaspoons of Cider Vinegar, mix in a glass. Add very warm water and gargle.

GARGLE II: Mix 2 drops CLARY SAGE, 2 drops LAVENDER or ROSE GERANIUM and 1 drop CLOVE with ½ teaspoon of salt. Add 1 Cup of very warm water and gargle.

GARGLE III: Use 5 drops LEMON mixed in a cup of warm water.

FEVER

ESSENTIAL OILS IN THIS SECTION: LEMON, LEMONGRASS, PALMAROSA, LIME, PEPPERMINT.

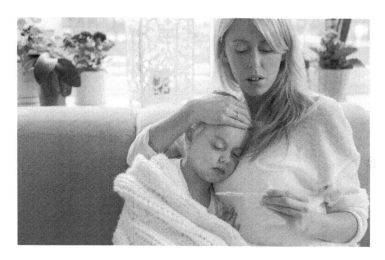

Fever is one of the ways the body reacts to defend itself. A temperature of 102-104, according to experts, can help shorten an infection. However a high temper, or one that continues for more time, can be dangerous and may need a doctor's attention.

Some ways to help bring down a fever if needed are:

LEMON essential oil can help bring down fever and relieve symptoms of flu. Diffuse it, blend 10 drops in an ounce of cream and massage to the body; use a cold compress after swishing it in 10 drops of lemon; put 10 drops in a cool bath.

BRING DOWN FEVER. LEMONGRASS helps brings down fever. In traditional medicine and in herbal medicine, LEMONGRASS is used to reduce fevers. It has a cooling effect,

73

and its anti-inflammatory actions also reduce heat. To use, blend with your basic carrier oil (10 drops in 1 ounce) and apply to the back of neck, chest area, and the bottom of feet. Also diffuse if running a fever, or inhale directly every 30-45 minutes.

LIME has qualities to help down fever. Inhale, put on cold compress, put in a cold bath.

PALMAROSA is another essential oil that has traditionally helped bring down fever. Use it the same way as above!

SPONGE BATH: A sponge bath can be helpful if one is too sick for a bath, or a bathtub is not available. Use 7-10 drops of any of the essential oils above, or PEPPERMINT, swish the sponge in the water, wring and use on the body to help bring relief.

INFLAMMATION OR STIFFNESS, ARTHRITIS, RHEUMATOID ARTHRITIS, RHEUMATISM

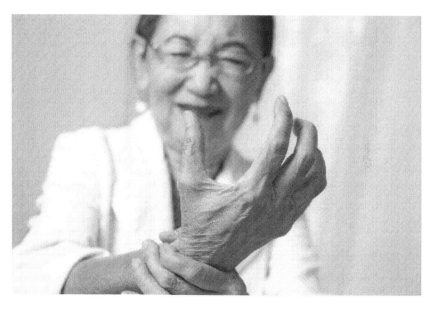

ESSENTIAL OILS USED IN THIS SECTION: TURMERIC, FRANKINCENSE, CEDARWOOD, LAVENDER, MAY CHANG, STAR ANISE, ROSE GERANIUM , SWEET ORANGE , BASIL, CLOVE, HELICHRYSUM

MY PERSONAL FAVORITES: Turmeric and Frankincense!

What is the difference between Rheumatism, Rheumatoid Arthritis and Arthritis?

Arthritis usually happens later in life and the pain caused is due to wear-and-tear on joints. Rheumatoid Arthritis can occur at any age, and is an auto-immune disease that affects the joints. Rheumatism is an older-fashioned term no longer used in medical dictionaries. It could be defined as any disease of inflammation that affects the joints!

Stiff or Arthritic Hands, Wrists, Knees: Use 4 drops LAVENDER and 4 drops FRANKINCENSE mixed into your favorite cream or oil, and massage on the area of stiffness or inflammation.

In the U.K., Cardiff University scientists found that FRANKINCENSE could inhibit the production of key inflammatory molecules, helping prevent the breakdown of the cartilage tissue that causes these conditions. (ScienceDaily August 4, 2011.) Put some 6-8 drops in an oil or organic cream, and rub topically on hands or joints daily or 4 times weekly.

ARTHRITIS INFLAMMATION: Use TURMERIC in an organic cream or oil (use any cream, or something like shea butter or coconut!) Use 10 drops per ounce

PAIN & INFLAMMATION: Inhale SWEET ORANGE, diffuse, add to bath water, or a compress. Orange blends well with LAVENDER & ROSE GERANIUM. Use about 10 drops per ounce if you are mixing into a cream or oil to help reduce inflammation or pain.

ANTI-INFLAMMATORY SOOTHER: HELICHRYSUM is a pain reliever with anti-inflammatory powers. Mix 10 drops along with 8 drops of LAVENDER in an ounce of carrier, massage on frequently.

INFLAMMATION OF THE FACE: Use ROSE GERANIUM in a small jar of your favorite face cream or serum. It helps with inflammation, promotes circulation (great for skin tone), and has great qualities for skin and body systems. Use it after a late night out!

ACHY MUSCLES? The pain-relieving and anti-inflammatory qualities of BASIL can help. Put 6-7 drops in a cream and massage on those achy muscles. You could also blend in ROSE GERANIUM or CLARY SAGE (4 drops of Basil to 3 drops of the other.)

SOAK IN A WARM TO HOT BATH: Add 10 drops of your favorite essential oil listed. Clove is very warming to the joints and can help (but don't use this if you are on a blood thinner, nor Turmeric.)

WARM COMPRESS: This is especially good for stiff and painful fingers, hands, wrists or knee. Use 5 drops of FRANKINCENSE and 5 drops of TURMERIC or LAVENDER in a bowl of warm water, swish your compress, wring it out and apply.

TOPICAL WITH EASTERN INFLUENCE: Blend 4 drops of MAY CHANG to 20 drops of coconut oil and apply to skin – it can help relieve pain, muscular tension, respiratory ailments, arthritis and rheumatism.

ROSEMARY and/or FRANKINCENSE before or after your yoga or exercise session can help with muscular pain (or preventing it!

A PREMADE TOPICAL: Our Zen DeStress Topical Blend does wonders for tight muscles or tension (in the shoulders, legs, etc.) The blend is LAVENDER, CLARY SAGE, NEROLI, ROMAN

CHAMOMILE & ROSEMARY in organic sunflower & jojoba.

DIGESTIVES ISSUES

INCLUDES UPSET TUMMY, INDIGESTION, IBS, NAUSEA, MOTION SICKNESS, SLUGGISH LIVER

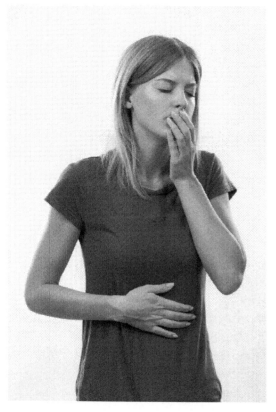

ESSENTIAL OILS IN THIS SECTION: PEPPERMINT, ORANGE, ROMAN CHAMOMILE, BERGAMOT, TURMERIC, STAR ANISE, LEMON, CLARY SAGE, SPEARMINT, CLOVE, NEROLI, SANDALWOOD, MAY

Upset stomach, nausea or motion sickness? Inhaling PEPPERMINT can eliminate the effects of nausea and motion sickness, simply because of its relaxing and soothing effects. In addition to inhaling, mix 5-7 drops PEPPERMINT in an ounce of carrier, and then apply directly on the forehead or rub on your stomach.

Chemotherapy-Induced Nausea: A 2013 study found that PEPPERMINT was found to be effective in reducing chemotherapy-induced nausea, and at reduced cost versus standard drug-based treatment (plus safer and more pleasant.)

Feeling nauseous and don't have Peppermint? LEMON can substitute in a pinch. A recent study showed that symptoms decreased after 2 days in 100 women who suffered nausea and used lemon essential oil. (Inhale deeply, and you can also mix 7 drops of LEMON in an ounce of cream and rub on your stomach.)

Aids Digestion. CLARY SAGE boosts the secretion of gastric juices and bile, which speeds up and eases the digestive process. By relieving symptoms of indigestion, it minimizes cramping, bloating and abdominal discomfort. This powerful essential oil also prevents stomach disorders and helps the body to absorb the much-needed vitamins and minerals that are consumed throughout the day. It regulates bowel movements, relieves constipation, and heals ulcer symptoms and wounds in the stomach.

Digestive support: SWEET ORANGE is one a good choice for digestive disorders. It reduces constipation, gas, abdominal spasms, nausea, and vomiting. It's also used for irritable bowel syndrome.

Here is a recipe for IBS:

5 drops Orange + 5 drops Roman Chamomile + 4 drops Bergamot + 5 drops Sandalwood
Bergamot is also known to help with abdominal cramps and digestive discomfort such as excess gas.

IBS? TURMERIC could help. Blend 6 drops it into an ounce of oil or cream and massage on your belly.

Ease Indigestion or IBS: Blend 4 drops SPEARMINT, 4 drops CLOVE, 2 drops NEROLI into 4 teaspoons of your carrier massage on your tummy.

More on IBS: Research has also shown that PEPPERMINT is effective in improving the symptoms of irritable bowel syndrome (IBS). It has helped reduce the total irritable bowel syndrome score by 50 percent among 75 percent of the participants of a specific study. Use it in various ways: mix 12 drops in a carrier and massage on the stomach; inhale often; use it in a bath or soak; put a warm compress (10 drops in bowl of water) and use on your lower stomach.

Indigestion? In China and other East Asian countries, STAR ANISE is used for problems such as bloating, abdominal cramps, gas, indigestion and constipation and also activates the metabolic enzymes. Put 5 drops in a carrier and massage on; inhale or diffuse. It blends well with Peppermint - use 2 drops of each.

Indigestion: We tend to think of Peppermint in the West as the top essential oil for indigestion, but LEMONGRASS has been used for centuries for this condition. Inhale deeply; you can also put 6 drops in an ounce of a carrier, and massage on your tummy.

Vomiting or nauseous indigestion: First, not everyone likes the aroma of PEPPERMINT, more often thought of for this use. If this is the case, use BASIL. Diffuse, inhale, mix 5-7 drops in an ounce of carrier and rub on your tummy.

Sluggish Digestion? TURMERIC can help with liver congestion, cleansing and sluggish digestion in moderation and in short bouts – use it in an oil or cream and massage on your mid-section at a higher dilution that normal (10 drops +/-).

Gas. BERGAMOT helps with excess gas and abdominal cramps. Inhale, diffuse, put 5-6 drops in an ounce and massage on mid-section.

More gas: MAY CHANG has long been used in traditional Chinese medicine to treat gas. Put 5-6 drops in your body cream or oil and massage on your tummy when the problem occurs + inhale. Repeat every few hours as needed.

Gas or nervous stomach? PETITGRAIN helps with gas or nervous stomach. Put 5 drops in your body cream or in a carrier oil and rub on your tummy for relief. Also inhale it before and after topical application.

INSOMNIA, PROBLEMS WITH SLEEP

ESSENTIAL OILS IN THIS SECTION: LAVENDER, CLARY SAGE, ROMAN CHAMOMILE

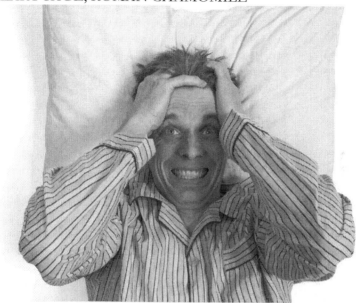

LAVENDER is the top essential oil for insomnia. Diffuse it in your bedroom at night; inhale it; apply it topically in a cream (7-10 drops per ounce.) CLARY SAGE is also a sedative and works very well with LAVENDER.

PREMADE TOPICAL: Our SUBLIME SLEEP topical blend with LAVENDER, CLARY SAGE and other essential oils helps slow the mind and relax the body. This is especially good to use if you WAKE UP in the night and your mind is racing. You can also apply this at night while diffusing LAVENDER.

BEDTIME BATH: ROMAN CHAMOMILE and LAVENDER

is a good mix to use in a soothing, warm bath before bed.

CUTS - BURNS

ESSENTIAL OILS IN THIS SECTION: LAVENDER, ROSE GERANIUM, TURMERIC, FRANKINCENSE, TEA TREE, HELICHRYSUM

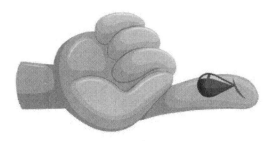

LAVENDER is renowned for its ability to heal the skin (burns, ulcers, rashes, irritations, infections, wounds, and other types of damage) and can be used "neat". I keep a bottle in the kitchen!

FRANKINCENSE could also be used directly (after a patch test) for new scrapes, cuts or boils to disinfect and help heal.

ROSE GERANIUM (after that patch test!) can be applied directly to heal cuts & wounds. This is a good choice if the cut continues to bleed, as it speeds up clotting.

A BLEND FOR A CUT OR WOUND: Blend 4 drops of TURMERIC with 5 drops LAVENDER and apply directly to your cut or wound to help disinfect and heal.

HELICHRYSUM works well for burns (and scars from burns). After a patch test, you could apply this neat in the first few days. After blend 7-10 drops in an ounce of jojoba or baobab oil.

Finally TEA TREE is another choice for your cut or wound (after patch test) to disinfect.

STREP, STAPH, MRSA, ANTI-BACTERIALS

ESSENTIAL OILS IN THIS SECTION: LAVENDER, TEA TREE, EUCALYPTUS, CLARY SAGE, CINNAMON, CLOVE, LEMON, LEMONGRASS, ROSEMARY, THYME, CEDARWOOD, STAR ANISE, OREGANO, BASIL

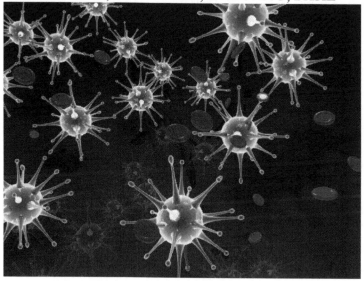

Note that most essential oils have anti-bacterial qualities. However, some excel at this due to their components, and we focus on these here.

My favorite study showing the powers of essential oils was done in the south of France: 210 colonies of bacteria & microbes were grown in petri dishes. Essential oils were then diffused into the air of these colonies - and all except 3 colonies were entirely wiped out in 20 minutes! The remaining 3 were dead within an hour. (I write about this in more detail in my book "Essential Oils Have Super Powers.")

TEA TREE was one of the essential oils used in a live hospital case to kill MRSA (Methicillin-Resistant Staphylococcus Aureus also known as an antibiotic-resistant superbug.) The doctor was able to save a man's leg from amputation. Dr. Eugene Sherry at the University of Sydney in Australia used a solution of tea tree and eucalyptus on the deep leg wound over a period of 3 weeks after all hope had been lost.

In another MRSA case, CINNAMON BARK was used to eradicate a MRSA infection and avoid amputation.

Cornell Research: Researchers at Cornell University found that a combination of LAVENDER, ROSE GERANIUM and TEA TREE were able to inhibit the growth of antibiotic-resistant bacteria.

Hospital Study: As we wrote earlier, researchers at Australia's Royal Brisbane and Women's Hospital found that TEA TREE, EUCALYPTUS and LEMONGRASS inhibited bacteria in large measure, notably higher and better than rubbing alcohol. They also tested the essential oils against the most deadly of the superbugs and found them to be highly effective.

Superior: OREGANO is one of the strongest anti-bacterials, thanks to strong components such as carvacrol and thymol. Many believe OREGANO is one of the best. A team of British and Indian doctors tested it and found it kills MRSA. Diffuse it! Use in a throat cream (6 drops to an ounce.) A tent steam is an excellent way to hone in on those bacteria.

Antibacterial: CEDARWOOD essential oil can be applied

topically on wounds as an antiseptic (typically blended with coconut oil, an organic gel, or if direct, do your patch test first.) It defends the body against toxins and relieves your white blood cells and immune system of stress or malfunction — this protects your internal functions and fights off bacteria in the body. Create a blend by mixing 10-12 drops of CEDARWOOD essential oil with an ounce of coconut oil, and then rub the mixture on your body to help with wounds or infections.

FOUR THIEVES! Do you know the story of the 4 thieves of Marseilles, during the medieval Black Death or Plague in Europe? These men doused themselves with essential oils and aromatic plants, and were able to rob the dead victims of the Plague without ever becoming ill, The Plague had a very high mortality rate. (We use the same blend in our ZEN IMMUNE BOOST!)

A doctor did a test on the same blend in a diffusion: he diffused EUCALYPTUS, CLOVE, ROSEMARY, CINNAMON and LEMON in a room with various bacterial cultures. It reduced all of the bacteria significantly within 10 minutes.

Anti-Staphylococcal! A 2015 study published in Postepy Dermatol Alergol Journal found that CLARY SAGE essential oil may be effectively applied to treat wounds and skin infections due to its antimicrobial properties. It indicated a strong anti-staphylococcal activity against clinical strains isolated from wound infections — the oil was active against strains, including Staphylococcus aureus, S. epidermidis and S. xylosus.

Effective Against 67 Strains: Researchers in Taiwan tested four new antimicrobial compounds from STAR ANISE and found that they were effective against 67 strains of drug-resistant bacteria. Published in the October 2010 issue of "Journal of Medicinal Food," the researchers reported that their findings pave the way for the development of new antibiotic medicines.

Anti-bacterial Study: A study published in BIOMED CENTRAL ("In vitro antibacterial activity of some plant essential oils", 2006) concluded after testing a number of essential oils on strong bacteria that CINNAMON, CLOVE, & LIME were found to inhibit both gram-positive and gram-negative bacteria (the others tested tended to inhibit one or the other)

Staph Killer: LEMONGRASS is very effective against staph infections in clinical tests. Diffuse or use 10 drops to an ounce of a carrier and apply.

BITES OR STINGS, RASHES, ITCHY SKIN

ESSENTIAL OILS IN THIS SECTION: LAVENDER, PEPPERMINT, CLARY SAGE

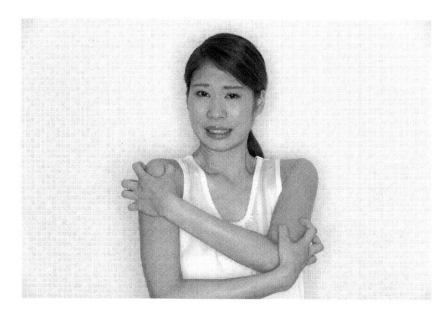

My personal favorite for mosquito bites (common in Florida) is Peppermint!

Irritations. LAVENDER can help with irritations and bites.

Itchy Mosquito or Fire Ant Bites? Thanks to the cooling menthol sensation in PEPPERMINT, a few drops can relieve the itch.

Rashes. CLARY SAGE is known to help with rashes, plus it helps regulate production of oil on the skin. Blend Clary (about 5-6 drops) in an ounce of jojoba or your favorite cream and apply.

☐

LOSS OF APPETITE

ESSENTIAL OILS IN THIS SECTION: LEMONGRASS, BERGAMOT, SPEARMINT

Loss of Appetite? The scent of Lemongrass, a culinary herb used in Asian cuisine, has appetite-stimulating properties. Inhale if bored with food or if you have no appetite.

BERGAMOT or SPEARMINT may also help with appetite.

WOMEN'S ISSUES

ESSENTIAL OILS IN THIS SECTION: CLARY SAGE, PETIT GRAIN, LEMONGRASS, YLANG YLANG, MARJORAM, SANDALWOOD, FENNEL

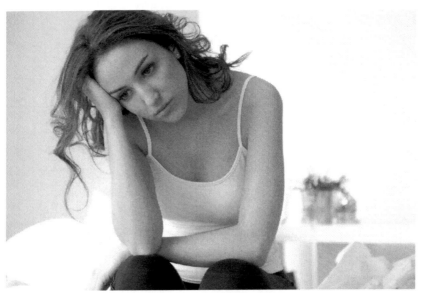

CLARY SAGE is considered to be the top women's essential oil.

Cramps, menstrual issues, hormonal imbalance or other related issues? Many health issues today, even things like infertility, polycystic ovary syndrome and estrogen-based cancers, are caused from <u>excess estrogen</u> in the body — in part because of our consumption of high-estrogen foods. Because CLARY SAGE helps balance out those estrogen levels, it's an incredibly effective essential oil. Create a massage oil by diluting 5 drops of clary sage oil with 5 drops of a carrier oil (like jojoba or coconut oil) and apply it to needed areas. If you have a bad case of cramps, inhale or diffuse as well.

Cramps or spasms? PETITGRAIN has qualities that are anti-spasmodic. If suffering from cramps or spasms, inhale Petitgrain or diffuse it, then add several drops to an oil or cream and massage in the area of the cramps. It induces relaxation in the tissues, muscles, nerves, and blood vessels. Repeat every few hours if necessary.

Ease Menstrual Cramps: In Eastern medicine, LEMONGRASS is used to ease cramps. (CLARY SAGE is most used in the West.) If suffering from cramps, inhale every 30 minutes + put 6-10 drops in an ounce of carrier and massage on your lower abdomen.

For PMS: Blend 6 drops YLANG YLANG (and if you wish, add 2 drops LAVENDER) in 1 ounce of a carrier oil or cream and apply to the back of neck and lower abdomen to help relieve symptoms.

PMS II: Here is another blend to try for several PMS 4 drops MAJORAM, 4 drops SANDALWOOD, 2 drops CLARY SAGE & 1 drop FENNEL on your abdomen, and also inhale the scents.

ORAL HEALTH

ESSENTIAL OILS USED IN THIS SECTION: TEA TREE, PEPPERMINT, CLOVE

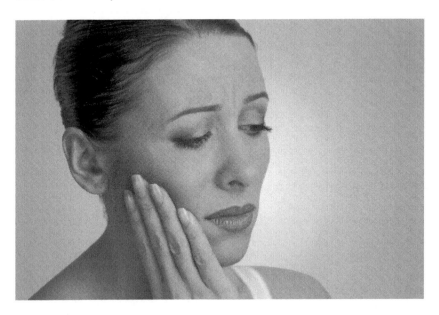

Oral health is directly related to overall health.

TEA TREE is known to fight oral candidiasis, prevent gum disease and help prevent sore throats. Put a drop on your toothpaste, or put a drop in your organic oil for oil pulling to swish in your mouth (I do this from time to time in my Sesame oil, though more often with PEPPERMINT). You can also put a few drops in warm water and gargle if you feel a sore throat coming on.

PEPPERMINT has been found to be superior to the mouthwash chemical chlorhexidine inhibiting Streptococus Mutans-driven biofilm formation associated with dental caries. It also helps reduce bacteria that causes bad breath.

Tooth ache? Dip a Q-tip into a little CLOVE, and touch it on the affected area. This will help relieve inflammation, be an antiseptic against bacteria and pain reliever.

Pain Relief Study: In one study published in The Journal of Dentistry in 2006 (there have been many other studies), a team of dentists recruited 73 adult volunteers and randomly split them into groups that had one of four substances applied to the gums just next to the canine tooth: a CLOVE (in a gel), benzocaine, a placebo resembling the CLOVE, or a placebo resembling benzocaine. Then, after five minutes, they compared what happened when the subjects received two needle sticks in those areas. Not surprisingly, the placebos failed to numb the tissue against the pain, but the CLOVE and benzocaine applications numbed the tissue equally well. "No significant difference was observed between CLOVE and benzocaine regarding pain scores," the scientists concluded.

Toothpaste Recipe: Put 6 tablespoons of organic coconut oil (or sesame oil) to 6 tablespoons of baking soda, mix in a container that seals or closes well; then add 10-15 drops of CLOVE essential oil (or if you prefer, use PEPPERMINT instead).

SWOLLEN ANKLES, ACHING FEET

ESSENTIAL OILS IN THIS SECTION: PEPPERMINT, ROSE GERANIUM, TURMERIC, EUCALYPTUS, LAVENDER

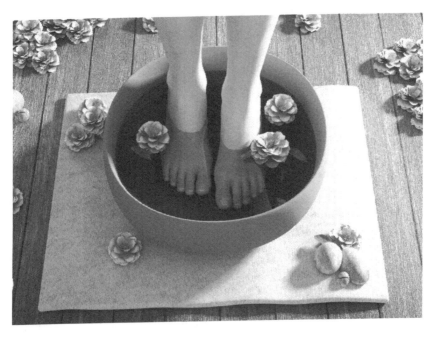

Tired, achy feet? Soak your feet in water with PEPPERMINT. It's refreshing and invigorating! Use about 6 drops.

Refreshing spray. You can also create a refreshing spray for your feet and lower legs. Using a 4 ounce spray bottle, mix 30 drops of Peppermint in 1 teaspoon of vodka then top off the 4 oz bottle with distilled water. Always shake before use (water and oil will separate, but water is the carrier. Shaking before use mixes it again.) Mist your feet, ankles and lower legs – it is refreshing and helps revive! It could be good in the summer for refreshing your hot feet, too! (<u>Keep this in the fridge</u>.)

Swollen ankles? ROSE GERANIUM can be used in a nice cool foot soak to help reduce the inflammation. (You could also add 4-5 drops to your body cream or oil and massage on your feet, ankles and calves.)

Bath or Foot Bath. After a long day or week, put a few drops of EUCALYPTUS in your bath, or do a foot soak. You will feel revived and breathe clearer! This is especially good on a weeknight when you have to get up for work or school the next day – it helps revive and fortify you.

POOR CIRCULATION

ESSENTIAL OILS USED IN THIS SECTION: LEMON, CLARY SAGE, CINNAMON, BASIL, BLACK PEPPER.

LEMON is very beneficial to circulation! It can help with varicose veins, help with sluggish systems and blocked energy.

Increases Circulation. CLARY SAGE opens the blood vessels and allows for increased blood circulation; it also naturally lowers blood pressure by relaxing the brain and arteries. This can boost the performance of the metabolic system by increasing the amount of oxygen that gets into the muscles and supporting organ function.

Topical Circulation Boost Blend (premade). Our Circulation Boost Blend is mixed in Jojoba & Sunflower with GINGER: Well known for anti-inflammatory powers as well as support of the immune system, helping with circulation and reducing pain.

CINNAMON: One of my favorites, a warming essential oil. It decreases inflammation, fights free radicals, warms the body, stimulates the immune system and can dilute blood vessels.

ROSEMARY: Is stimulating to mind and soul, energizes and uplifts. Promotes cognitive alertness, and helps the body with regeneration, circulation and fatigue.

BASIL: Helpful antioxidant, which helps guard against degeneration and enhances well-being. Basil is known to be anti-spasmodic .

Cold limbs due to poor circulation issues? If your feet and/or hands are cold – due to weather or due to circulatory issues - you can use CINNAMON in several ways. Have a warm foot soak prepared, put 3-5 drops in a warm bath! You can put 4 drops in your favorite cream or oil, and massage your feet, legs and hands to help stimulate circulation and warmth. (Skin Brushing before will also help – see www.skin-brushing.com)

URINARY TRACT INFECTION

ESSENTIAL OILS USED IN THIS SECTION:
BERGAMOT

The Journal of Applied Microbiology published that BERGAMOT produced positive results against Enterococcus faecium and Enterococcus faecalis bacteria, potent antibiotic-resistant microbes. These enterococcal species are a common source of a variety of infections, including urinary tract infections (UTI), bacteremia, endocarditis, and meningitis.

Sitz Bath: Add 6 to 8 drop of BERGAMOT essential oil to your sitz bath or hip bath to help prevent the spread of bacterial infections from the urethra into the bladder. It has shown great effectiveness against the specific bacteria that causes these infections.

In addition, make a topical with 10-12 drops of BERGAMOT in a carrier oil, and massage on lower abdomen.

OREGANO may also help as it is a strong bactericide. Add some to your sitz bath; make a topical with 7-8 drops to massage on.

REPEL PESTS

ESSENTIAL OILS USED IN THIS SECTION:
LAVENDER, PEPPERMINT, CLOVE, CEDARWOOD,
LEMON, LEMONGRASS

Scorpions, Insects. LAVENDER is the "go-to" to repel scorpions. It can work on other insects as well.

Insects, Ants or Mice in the house? Put 4-5 drops of PEPPERMINT on a tea bag or cotton ball, and place at the back of kitchen cabinets or where there may be holes in the wall or cabinets (points of entry) as a deterrent.

Spiders, Bugs. CLOVE can repel spiders and bugs. Dot it around the home on cotton balls or tea bags; diffuse.

Mosquitos. This is a tough one. Why? The best mosquito repellents are the citrus essential oils like LEMON & LEMONGRASS but they are PHOTO-TOXIC, so you can't use them on your skin during the day! That is, you can't put them on your skin (mixed in a carrier) and go into the sun, or you will burn. So during daytime, dot them on your clothing, put them on your aromatherapy jewelry (necklace, bracelet). Use while hiking or camping, in the tent, dot on your socks, hat, backpack and clothing.

Otherwise, use the non-citrus oils in skin lotions (like CINNAMON, CEDARWOOD, PEPPERMINT.) Small diffusers that run on USB cables are helpful in camping or outdoor situations. Of course, you can diffuse LEMON or LEMONGRASS on your patio, porch or in the home.

For your topical, mix 6-8 drops of the chosen oil into your cream, oil or gel.

Moths, Insects. CEDARWOOD was originally used in chests and storage boxes thanks to the repellent nature of the wood, to protect contents of the box from critters. It has been found to repel all sorts of insects, including mosquitos.

Insect Repellent. Insects hate the smell of CINNAMON. Diffuse it; use it in the home (back of cabinets for instance), or blended in a topical cream for use on your skin while outdoors. It is not photo-toxic like the citrus oils and you could consider using in warmer climates or during the summer to scare away insects.

POST VIRAL RECOVERY

ESSENTIAL OILS USED IN THIS SECTION: TURMERIC, MAY CHANG, CARDAMON

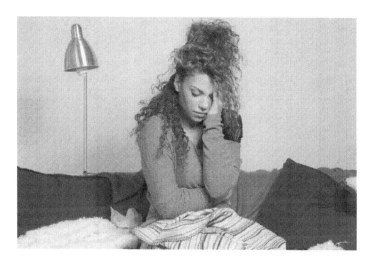

Getting over a Viral Infection or Bout? TURMERIC has been shown to help in the recovery from a viral infection. Use it in a massage (6 drops in an ounce), and/or use it in a soak or bath.

Post Viral Recovery Recipe for a Bath: 3 drops MAY CHANG and 5 drops CARDAMON in a bath. Apply to warm or hot water or put on bath salts.

SHINGLES/ POST RECOVERY

ESSENTIAL OILS USED IN THIS SECTION:
PEPPERMINT, PALMAROSA

Shingles Associated Pain (Post-Herpetic Neuralgia): A 2002 case study found that topical PEPPERMINT treatment resulted in a near immediate improvement of shingles associated neuropathic pain symptoms; the therapeutic effects persisted throughout the entire 2 months of follow-up treatment. Use a higher dosage (say 10-12 drops) in your organic oil, cream or gel; diffuse.

PALMAROSA is an essential oil that can help in the recovery from – or even help reduce – shingles.

FAST HEARTBEAT

ESSENTIAL OILS USED IN THIS SECTION: YLANG YLANG, MAY CHANG, LAVENDER, ROSEMARY

YLANG YLANG is considered to be a very sensual oil, euphoric and, of course, romantic. But it is also considered to be soothing to the heart. The French chemists Garnier and Rechler first recognized this medicinal property of YLANG YLANG and its calming effect on the heart during times of distress (slowing a racing heart, helping to reduce stress.) Inhale immediately if experiencing a fast heartbeat; use a body cream with 5-7 drops per ounce if you have a propensity. You can also add 2 drops of Lavender to your topical or inhaler.

Not that in Chinese medicine, YLANG YLANG's calming effect on the heart is its primary therapeutic action.

Scientific study. Robert Tisserand wrote in a scientific study that May Chang (Litsea Cubeba) can help control arrhythmia (which is a common sign of stress and anxiety) and induce relaxation.

Calming. Rosemary brings down cortisol levels, which rise during stress, and could be used to help calm a fast-beating heart. Inhale it at once!

FUNGAL INFECTIONS - MOLD

ESSENTIAL OILS USED IN THIS SECTION: TEA TREE, MAY CHANG, CLOVE, GINGER, OREGANO, BERGAMOT

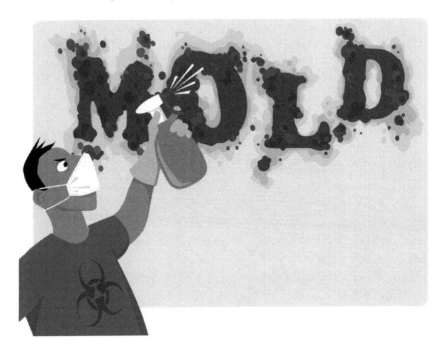

Anti-fungal and anti-bacterial in your environment. Diffuse TEA TREE (and inhale it) when you wish to bring extra force to clearing microbes.

AC ducts. TEA TREE is a good essential oil to use in your air conditioning filters, to help keep fungi out of ducts. Simply put a few drops on the filter and/or in the ducts.

Moldy basement? If you have a moldy basement, diffuse TEA

TREE to take care of the situation (you could add a few drops of LAVENDER or ROSE GERANIUM if the scent it too medicinal for you.)

I wrote about embarrassing fungal-based issues like athlete's foot, jock itch and fungal infections of the toenail in the second chapter of this book, under TEA TREE. Do refer to that section!

Candida. In a study published in the Journal of Antimicrobial Chemotherapy, Italian researchers have proven BERGAMOT essential oil's amazing antifungal properties when used as a topical remedy for infections brought by candida fungus strains. Blend 6-7 drops of BERGAMOT into an ounce and massage on your abdomen; inhale or diffuse.

Fungus and mold in damp hidden areas (inside of your washing machine liner, the shower corner?) Put some TEA TREE on a cloth and wipe down the area. Add a drop of LEMON for extra anti-bacterial action and a touch of freshness. I like to do this in drains, too!

Stinky shoes? Mix 10 drops of TEA TREE in baking soda (you can also add a few drops of PEPPERMINT or LAVENDER), sprinkle in your shoes, let them sit overnight and then shake them out the next morning.

Fungal power. Though we tend to use TEA TREE to attack fungus, TURMERIC has been shown to have excellent powers in this area and is commonly used in the East for this.

You can use MAY CHANG for fungus or mold, or combine MAY CHANG and TEA TREE (some like the scent of the 2 together better than just TEA TREE.) Diffuse together in moldy areas; use in your bathroom corners.

109

RESTLESS LEG SYNDROME

ESSENTIAL OIL USED IN THIS SECTION: BERGAMOT

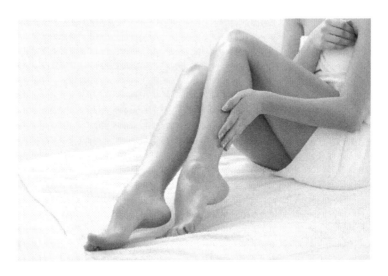

Restless Leg Syndrome or Muscle Tensions? BERGAMOT could help! Put about 15 drops in a carrier oil and massage your legs.

SORE MUSCLES

ESSENTIAL OILS USED IN THIS SECTION: CLOVE, EUCALYPTUS, BERGAMOT, FRANKINCENSE, ROSE GERANIUM, TURMERIC, MAY CHANG, CLARY SAGE, BASIL, VETIVER, WINTERGREEN, GINGER, BLUE CHAMOMILE

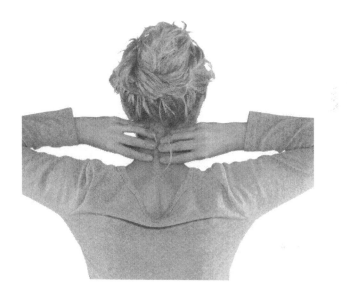

Tight muscles, bad pain in legs or shoulders? CLOVE & TURMERIC can help you. Use in a warm compress, bath soak, or do a body gel with 4 drops each in an ounce.

Sore, fatigued muscles? EUCALYPTUS is great to help revive you. Inhale or diffuse - plus if you have muscular tiredness, you can put 4-6 drops in your favorite oil or cream and massage to set yourself right.

Back pain or muscular woes? Traditional Chinese medicine uses MAY CHANG to treat these conditions. Do a compress (warm or cold) with MAY CHANG to bring down inflammation and pain. (Put 4-6 drops in the water, swish your wash cloth, wring and place on the area. Be sure not to get it in your eyes.)

You can also combine TURMERIC or FRANKINCENSE in your compress for muscular pains. Likewise, 3 drops of MAY CHANG blended with 20 drops of coconut oil and apply to skin – it can help relieve pain, headache, muscular tension, respiratory ailments, arthritis and rheumatism.

Exercise sore? Use FRANKINCENSE and/or ROSEMARY to relieve the soreness all over. You could also apply your body lotion BEFORE you exercise! Use a total of 8 drops of your choice in an ounce of gel, oil or cream and massage on.

Achy muscles? The pain-relieving and anti-inflammatory qualities of BASIL can help. Put 6-7 drops in a cream and massage on those achy muscles.

Muscle Relief: You could also blend ROSE GERANIUM or CLARY SAGE with BASIL (3-4 drops of Basil to 2 drops of the others) for a nice body topical.

Pre-made blend: Our SORE MUSCLE BLEND is a topical and what I call the natural "icy hot". Blended in jojoba and sunflower, it includes:

WINTERGREEN - an excellent analgesic, good for arthritis and muscle pains. It's the active ingredient in methyl salicylate!
ROSEMARY - helps bring down stress and tension
ORGANIC BLUE CHAMOMILE - relaxes and soothes body and spirit

BLACK PEPPER - analgesic, anti-inflammatory
VETIVER - anti-inflammatory and sedative, helps bring down pain
GINGER - wonderful anti-inflammatory
BASIL - pain relieving qualities

AGE SPOTS

ESSENTIAL OILS USED IN THIS SECTION: MAY CHANG, LEMON, NEROLI, ROSE GERANIUM, ROMAN CHAMOMILE

MAY CHANG and LEMON have qualities that help lighten spots and are calming to skin. We devised an organic blend that includes other essential oils to help, the Age Spot Reducer, which includes:

LITSEA CUBEBA (MAY CHANG) - Calming, anti-inflammatory and antiseptic properties. Helpful to support reduction of age spots.
LEMON – Helps to actively lighten age spots. Penetrating and anti-inflammatory. However, lemon is photo-toxic – that is, you can't use lemon and go into the sun.
NEROLI – Contains citrol, which helps cell regeneration (new cells to help overcome age spots) and supports skin. Help tone and stabilize skin and has skin healing abilities.
ROSE GERANIUM – Helps normalize sebum in the skin and helps diminish age spots while keeping skin elastic. Improves blood circulation where it is applied. Excellent anti-aging essential oil.
ROMAN CHAMOMILE - Wonderful and soothing tonic for skin.
VITAMIN E oil – helpful oil for skin and in the process of reducing age spots.
Blended in organic jojoba and sunflower oils

STRETCH MARKS - SCARS

ESSENTIAL OILS USED IN THIS SECTION: ROSE GERANIUM, HELICHRYSUM, FRANKINCENSE, ROSEWOOD, LAVENDER

Scars, stretch marks or lines on your skin? ROSE GERANIUM is a powerful cicatrisant (that is, helps the fading of scars, marks and issues on the skin). It increases blood circulation just below the skin (which helps with healing and skin tone).

Put 10 drops in 1 ounce of a carrier and apply 3 times daily. We find Baobab Oil the best for this purpose since Baobab is also known as a scar reducer. Other oils like Jojoba would be perfectly fine!

Stretch marks from pregnancy? Blend 4 drops each of LAVENDER, FRANKINCENSE AND ROSEWOOD into ¼ cup of Rosehip Seed Oil (or Almond oil) and add a dash of Vitamin E oil.

Scar treatment. Try HELICHRYSUM neat (after a patch test), by applying a few drops up to 3 times daily on the scar and massaging.

114

ECZEMA, DERMATITIS, PSORIASIS

ESSENTIAL OILS USED IN THIS SECTION:
CEDARWOOD, PALMAROSA, TEA TREE, LAVENDER,
ROSE GERANIUM, ROSEWOOD, ROSEMARY, THYME,
CHAMOMILE, MYRRH, HELICHRYSUM, CAJUPUT, SAGE,
MANUKA, PATCHOULI, TURMERIC

Eczema. Eczema is a common skin disorder that causes dry, red,
itchy skin that can blister or crack. CEDARWOOD essential oil
can help reduce the inflammation that leads to this irritating skin
issue; it can help reduce skin peeling. Add 5-7 drops to 1 ounce of
your skin lotion, oil or cream and massage on the area; or put 5-10
drops in your bath and have a soak.

Eczema, dermatitis or psoriasis? Mix 10 drops of TEA TREE
with 5 drops of LAVENDER into an ounce of baobab or coconut
oil and apply twice daily or as needed.

Also could help eczema: BERGAMOT, CHAMOMILE, ROSE
GERANIUM, HELICHRYSUM, LAVENDER, MYRRH,
PALMAROSA, ROSEMARY and ROSEWOOD. Use any of these
(7-10 drops) in a cool compress, 1 ounce of body lotion, or bath
soak.

Could help dermatitis: CHAMOMILE, ROSE GERANIUM,
HELICHRYSUM, PATCHOULI, SAGE, SPEARMINT,
THYME. Use any of these (7-10 drops) in a cool compress, body
lotion or bath soak.

Could help psoriasis: Mix 10 drops BERGAMOT, 10 drops
THYME, 10 drops CAJUPUT and 10 drops MANUKA essential

115

oils into ½ cup of Grapeseed, Sweet Almond or Jojoba oil. After you daily shower, apply to skin.

Use this soap. TURMERIC soap is said to help with many skin conditions. We have one here.

Dermatitis treatment: Put 3 drops of HELICHRYSUM and 3 drops of LAVENDER in 6 drops of carrier oil, massage on. Note that both of these essential oils could be applied neat, but an equal amount of a carrier makes it easy to blend and massage on skin.

ACNE

ESSENTIAL OILS USED IN THIS SECTION: TEA TREE,
PEPPERMINT, LEMON, MAY CHANG, CLOVE,
CEDARWOOD, ROSEMARY, ORANGE, GRAPEFRUIT

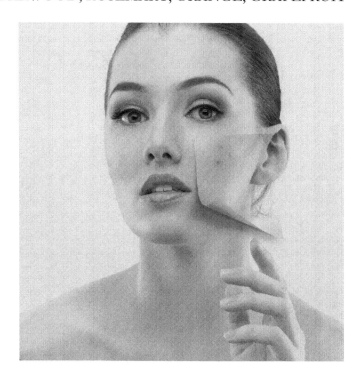

Breakouts, congested skin, oil or acne? Put 3 drops of PEPPERMINT in a steaming bowl of water and form a tent with a towel. Steam your face – then rinse with cool water. Make it a twice weekly regime.

Acne? TEA TREE can be used "neat" (direct drop without a carrier) on acne after your patch test. Otherwise, it works really well blended with jojoba oil or aloe gel. Blend about 15 drops in an ounce (a 3% dilution) and use twice daily.

Asian treatment. MAY CHANG has been long used in Asia for treating acne. Here are several ways to use it:
a) Do your patch test; if clear and no reactions, then use one drop directly on acne once per day.
b) Blend 6 drops MAY CHANG into an ounce of jojoba and use as your skin treatment
c) Blend 2 drops TEA TREE and 2-3 drop MAY CHANG into an ounce of witch hazel and a little water, shake well before applying and use as your astringent-acne treatment.
d) Do a steam tent with MAY CHANG to revive skin, clarify and help kill bacteria and oil on the skin.

Various studies have shown CLOVE is a good acne anti-bacterial. Put 3 drops CLOVE in 2 tablespoons of raw honey. Blend and apply. Let sit for at least 10 minutes, then wipe off; then rinse liberally with cool water and apply an astringent. Yes, it may be a little messy, but if you have bad acne, it is worth a try. The key is to not apply too much at one time – just dot a little on! You could also try a few drops in 2 tsp. of Jojoba instead.

Astringent. Add 2 drops of CEDARWOOD or TEA TREE to your toner for a nice tightening and refreshing feel. You can also do this by adding drops to organic jojoba or an organic aloe gel. CEDARWOOD can help with acne treatment, perhaps not as

118

common as tea tree. It helps tighten pores after cleansing them. Use a few drops in a cleanser or as mentioned above, as an astringent. You could also add 5 drops of CEDARWOOD to an ounce of coconut oil mixed with some oatmeal for a scrub.

Astringent. ROSEMARY is actually an astringent. Use it if you have oily skin or hair – put a few drops in your shampoo or cleansing toner.

Citrus Astringent. Many citrus oils, especially LEMON, MAY CHANG, GRAPEFRUIT and SWEET ORANGE, can tone the skin and reduce secretions. It's a good one to drop into some witch hazel and lightly smooth on skin with a cotton ball.

☐

ANTI-AGING SKIN CARE

ESSENTIAL OILS IN THIS SECTION: FRANKINCENSE, ROSE GERANIUM, NEROLI,

Cell regeneration. FRANKINCENSE is great as it encourages cell regeneration. Put 5-7 drops in an ounce of facial cream. I also love the scent, and put some FRANKINCENSE in a body oil that I use occasionally.

Anti-aging. ROSE GERANIUM is another essential oil great for aging skin. It helps with inflammation, promotes circulation (great for skin tone), and has helpful qualities for skin and body systems. I love to use it after a late night out! It can also relieve excessive dryness or help aging skin that is dry, works on wrinkles and helps reduce inflammation.

Healing. LAVENDER is renowned for its ability to heal the skin (burns, ulcers, rashes, irritations, infections, wounds, and other types of damage) and is good for aging skin care.

Naturally healing, helps with dry skin. NEROLI is a wonderful skin care essential oil, especially good for aging skin. Like FRANKINCENSE, it helps cell regeneration and is anti-inflammatory. It also helps with dry skin, marks and smoothness. (I frankly LOVE the scent.)

HAIR RESTORATION

ESSENTIAL OILS IN THIS SECTION: CEDARWOOD, YLANG YLANG, LAVENDER, ROSEMARY

Hair loss. In France, CEDARWOOD is included in commercial shampoos and hair lotions for hair loss or alopecia. It can help stimulate the hair follicles and increase circulation to the scalp which can contribute to hair growth and slow hair loss. Herbalists and aromatherapists often recommend it often for this condition.

Some research indicates that CEDARWOOD blended with LAVENDER and ROSEMARY could also help improve hair growth and health, by massaging it in and letting sit for 30 minutes (diluted of course, most often in coconut oil) or adding it to your shampoo. Research shows improvement over a 7 month period with daily use.

Thickening. YLANG YLANG has been highly sought after for centuries for its natural thickening effect on hair and also its healing properties on the skin. Put a few drops in your shampoo, and in your night cream!

OILY HAIR OR DANDRUFF

ESSENTIAL OILS USED IN THIS SECTION: TEA TREE, LAVENDER

Oily hair. Put a few drops of TEA TREE in your shampoo (especially if you have oily skin, a dandruff issue or an itchy scalp). It helps cleanse, remove excess oils and soothes your scalp!

If you want to try a natural home-made shampoo, try mixing TEA TREE & LAVENDER in aloe vera gel and coconut milk – especially good for dandruff.

HEAD LICE

ESSENTIAL OIL USED IN THIS SECTION:
PEPPERMINT, TEA TREE, ROSE GERANIUM

Did your child get head lice?

1) **Pretreatment before shampoo**. Since TEA TREE can be applied neat (after a patch test), use this BEFORE THE SHAMPOO IN DRIED HAIR "neat". Massage drops onto your child's scalp, massage and let sit for 40 minutes! Then shampoo.
2) Add 7 drops of TEA TREE to the shampoo, or use 7 drops of PEPPERMINT or use 7 drops of ROSE GERANIUM in the shampoo and massage in well, let sit; then rinse.
3) Repeat again later in the day and every day as needed.

Each of these essential oils have the ability to kill the lice.
You may wish to diffuse ROSE GERANIUM in your child's bedroom at night (PEPPERMINT is too energizing, TEA TREE is not typically liked by kids.) Put a drop in the laundry or dryer sheet, too, when handling their pillowcases and sheets.

SUGAR ADDICTION – WEIGHT LOSS

ESSENTIAL OILS USED IN THIS SECTION:
GRAPEFRUIT, PEPPERMINT, CINNAMON, FENNEL,
CLOVE, BERGAMOT, LIME, LEMON, SWEET ORANGE

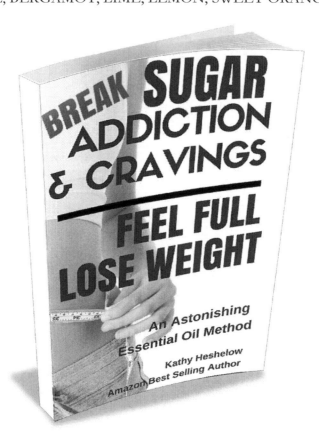

My Book Helps You Beat Sugar Addiction or Cravings (and Get on a Healthy Path with the help of Essential Oils. It also explains what sugar does to your satiety center, your addiction center and how it can encourage certain diseases – and offers a tested solution to help. It's found on Amazon here. I offer a free PEPPERMINT and 50% off GRAPEFRUIT & other recommended essential oils related to the book (offer found in the front of the book) while they last.

Study. The Journal of Psychoactive Drugs stated in a study published in 2010 that 'Sugar Addiction" follows the same pathways in the brain that a habit-forming drug does like morphine or heroine. In addition, too much sugar can help facilitate Candida yeast infections not to mention weight gain.

IMMUNE SYSTEM STRENGTH

ESSENTIAL OILS USED IN THIS SECTION:
FRANKINCENSE, EUCALPYTUS, CINNAMON, CLOVE,
OREGANO, ROSEMARY, LEMON, LEMONGRASS,
PEPPERMINT

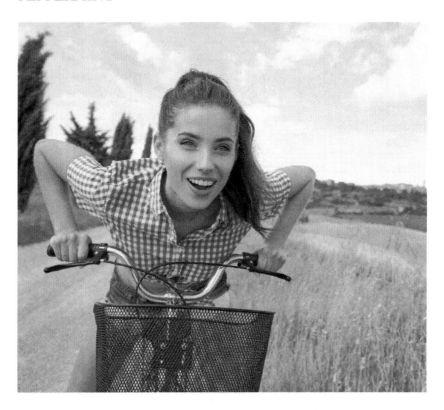

Essential oils can help support a healthy immune system and
wellness. Many essential oils have qualities that could be helpful in
some way for the immune system!

For this section, I refer to our pre-made blend called Immune

Boost, blended in jojoba and sunflower oils. Here are the oils and what they can do for the body:

EUCALYPTUS - well-known and multiple benefits, including sinus and respiratory applications, increases blood flow and help with mental exhaustion. (As early as the 1880s, surgeons were using eucalyptus oil as an antiseptic during operations.) According to a study published in recent BMC Immunology, eucalyptus oil extract is said to help the innate cell-mediated immune response.

OREGANO - strengthens and boosts the immune system, and stimulates function of the white blood cells. It is a truly powerful antimicrobial that can help fight off infections and parasites. It is known as a strong anti-fungal, too.

CINNAMON - helps to improve the circulation of blood which ensures oxygen supply to the body's cells, leading to a higher metabolic activity. Like clove, it can help clarify blood, too. Excellent energy booster and a great anti-bacterial.

CLOVE - able to purify blood and fight viruses. Antioxidants in this essential oil scavenge for dangerous free radicals. Strong anti-inflammatory and anti-bacterial. (It is often diffused in French clinics & hospitals against bacteria and microbes.)

ROSEMARY - has been proven to decrease the level of cortisol in the saliva. Cortisol is one of the main stress hormones, wearing you down and hurting the immune system. It is also a circulatory stimulant, helping the immune system.

LEMON - able to fight colds, flu and fatigue, the properties are great for immune boosting. It is an excellent astringent and is an antibacterial genius. Wonderful tonic for cleansing mind & body.

PEPPERMINT - one of the oldest European herbs used for

medicinal purposes, with historical accounts dating its use to ancient Chinese, Egyptian and Japanese folk medicine. Is healing and reviving. It has good antioxidant powers, and teamed up with its antimicrobial properties, this may help stimulate immune function.

FRANKINCENSE - also ancient in its uses (cited in the Bible, one of the highest used oils in ancient Mesopotamia and Sumer, well used in ancient Egypt), it promotes regeneration of healthy cells, helps bring down stress and anxiety for mental peace and relaxation, supports the immune system.

Immune stimulant: LEMONGRASS is rich in zinc, iron, calcium, potassium, magnesium, manganese, and sodium. These minerals are all important in the body's metabolic processes and the regulation of normal blood pressure and heart rate. It's recognized as an overall tonic! Diffuse it, inhale it!

Another great stimulant: Thanks to its high concentration of antiseptic organic compounds that stimulate the immune system and prevent dangerous infections, SIBERIAN FIR NEEDLE essential oil can be a powerful tool that keeps your body health inside and out.

STRESS, ANXIETY

ESSENTIAL OILS USED IN THIS SECTION: CLARY SAGE, ROSEMARY, LAVENDER, NEROLI, ORANGE, PETITGRAIN, LEMONGRASS

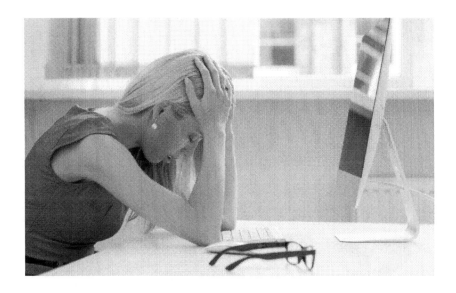

Stressed? If you feel highly stressed and cortisol levels are up, diffuse ROSEMARY or inhale it. Or add 7 drops to your favorite cream and massage on. You might put 2 drops on your aromatherapy bracelet or necklace and pull it close when you need to inhale.

Bring down cortisol levels. The Journal of Phytotherapy Research (2014) found that inhalation of CLARY SAGE essential oil had the ability to reduce cortisol levels by 36 percent and improved thyroid hormone levels. The study was done on 22 post-menopausal women in their 50s, some of whom were diagnosed with depression. At the end of the trial, the researchers stated that "CLARY SAGE had a statistically significant effect on lowering cortisol and had an anti-depressant effect improving mood."

LAVENDER is well known as a relaxant; it can help when you are stressed. Breathe it in deeply!

Nerve tonic. PETITGRAIN is famous as a nerve tonic (especially in France.) Soak in a bath (or soak feet at the end of the day) with 4-6 drops of PETITGRAIN. You can add 2 drops of LAVENDER if you wish! (French women love this!) Inhale whenever you feel the need.

Foot bath for stress: LEMONGRASS can be used in a bath or footbath to reduce stress. If you need some revival, use EUCALYPTUS.

Foot massage. Nothing is more relaxing that a foot massage to help bring down stress. Add several drops of LAVENDER or CLARY SAGE to the foot cream and enjoy!

Premade Topical. One of our most popular blends is called Zen De-Stress, and it is lovely! Put it on your pulse points as soon as you need it. The blend includes LAVENDER, CLARY SAGE, NEROLI, ROMAN CHAMOMILE AND ROSEMARY.

Note that this blend also works on physical stress – like tight shoulders or pain in the muscles. Apply directly.

DEPRESSION

ESSENTIAL OILS USED IN THIS SECTION: CLOVE, BERGAMOT, ROSEMARY, MAY CHANG, ROSE GERANIUM, LIME, PETIT GRAIN, BASIL, SWEET ORANGE

Feeling down, cold, depressed? The warmth of CLOVE along with its brightening qualities are excellent. Diffuse or inhale; use on your jewelry.

Anti-depressant. BERGAMOT is an anti-depressant and helps bring you out of the doldrums or grief. It is a happy scent that is bright and is great for emotional support. Diffuse it, inhale it, put 5-6 drops in your body cream!

Quite down, depressed and even stressed? ROSEMARY can help, since it brings down cortisol levels with stress, and is uplifting against your depression. Add 3-5 drops to your favorite cream and massage on. Inhale or diffuse. Use it in a bath at night.

Depressed and irritated? MAY CHANG is an anti-depressant. Diffuse it or inhale from the bottle or your own inhaler.

Need some uplift? SWEET ORANGE is an anti-depressant. It provides an uplifting and fresh feeling that it adds happiness to your life!

Nerve tonic. As mentioned earlier in the book, PETITGRAIN is famous as a nerve tonic. Soak in a bath (or soak feet at the end of the day) with 4-5 drops of Petitgrain.

Mental burnout and depression? BASIL is a good one to help overcome burnout and bring some uplift to you! Use it in a diffuser but also consider a nice BATH SOAK! Put BASIL in a soothing bath at the end of the day and relax.

Emotional balance needed? LIME helps emotional balance and well-being, and adds a sense of playfulness, appetite for life and zest for good. It helps release negativity and depression.

Mentally exhausted or depressed? Here are 2 applications to try; 1) Diffuse 2 drops CINNAMON and 4 drops SWEET ORANGE; 2) or put 2 drops of CINNAMON on a tissue, your aromatherapy jewelry or inhaler and inhale every 20 minutes.

Put a little Bliss in your life, premade blend. Another of our most favorite blends is Zen Air Bliss (not topical – this one is for the diffuser, or else blend it in a carrier for skin application). It includes:

YLANG YLANG - Encourages euphoria, relaxation and pleasure. Excellent against depression. Ideal to use in a massage oil.
SWEET ORANGE - Unblocks energy, combats pessimism and is bright and uplifting.
BERGAMOT - Restorative, helps reduce anxiety or worries, and is uplifting.
MAGNOLIA - Considered a sacred flower, revered in India for its relaxing and emotional confidence qualities.
NEROLI - Neroli is known to sooth nerves, facilitates creativity and calms the heart. It's also an aphrodisiac.

FATIGUE

ESSENTIAL OILS USED IN THIS SECTION:
EUCALYPTUS, BASIL, ROSE GERANIUM, CINNAMON,
SWEET ORANGE, FRANKINCENSE, CLARY SAGE

Tired, sore, fatigued? EUCALYPTUS is great to help revive you.
Inhale or diffuse - plus if you have muscular tiredness, you can put
a few drops in your favorite oil or cream and massage to set
yourself right. CLARY SAGE is also great for physical fatigue.

Mental Burnout? BASIL is one of the essential oils that can help
overcome burnout and bring some uplift! Use it in a diffuser but
also consider a nice bath soak or massage! Use 5 drops in an oil or
bath.

Fatigued? I love to use FRANKINCENSE in the diffuser.

Mental fatigue? ROSE GERANIUM, LAVENDER,
CINNAMON, ROSEMARY and PEPPERMINT all excel at
uplifting your mental fatigue. Choose one and diffuse or inhale it!
If you are going through a stretch of constant mental fatigue, make
a body blend with 5 drops of each essential oil into an ounce of a
carrier and apply morning and night.

General fatigue. LEMON could help! It's bright and happy.
Diffuse or inhale it!

GRIEF

ESSENTIAL OILS USED IN THIS SECTION: ROSE GERANIUM, LIME, LEMONGRASS

ROSE GERANIUM is known to be superior to help with grief and sadness. (It worked well for me after the death of a beloved pet.) Diffuse or inhale periodically during such a period. It is very balancing yet uplifting.

LIME or LEMONGRASS are anti-depressants and could help with emotional support.

TRANQUILITY

ESSENTIAL OILS USED IN THIS SECTION:
FRANKINCENSE, SWEET ORANGE, CLARY SAGE,
LAVENDER

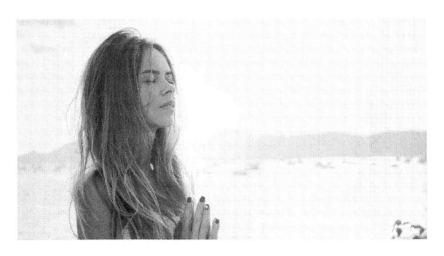

Tranquil environment. FRANKINCENSE is a perfect choice. It promotes a calm, tranquil setting. Diffuse or inhale.

Calm tranquility. CLARY SAGE or SWEET ORANGE also promote tranquility. Diffuse!

Blend for meditation or healing prayer. Mix 6 drops of CLARY SAGE with 2 drops of FRANKINCENSE or SWEET ORANGE. Diffuse!

You could also consider a body lotion using 2 drops of each in an ounce of carrier and apply before your meditation or prayers.

MEMORY

ESSENTIAL OIL USED IN THIS SECTION: ROSEMARY, BASIL, BLACK PEPPER

Clinical studies. Several recent clinical studies using ROSEMARY tested increase in memory, attentiveness, alertness, liveliness, and joyfulness, while increasing breathing rate and blood pressure. This confirms what herbalists and those through history have known (including Shakespeare!)

Researchers Moss and Oliver (2012) investigated plasma levels of 1,8 cineole after exposure to ROSEMARY, and it showed an increase of cognitive performance.

Diffuse it, inhale it, wear it on your aromatherapy jewelry; use it in a bath soak or foot soak; create a massage or body lotion with 6-7 drops of ROSEMARY to an ounce of a carrier. You could also add a drop of BASIL and/or BLACK PEPPER to this lotion.

APHRODISIAC

ESSENTIAL OILS USED IN THIS SECTION: YLANG YLANG, NEROLI, CLARY SAGE, STAR ANISE, CINNAMON, JASMINE, SANDALWOOD

MY PERSONAL FAVORITE: While I like YLANG YLANG, I prefer and adore NEROLI best!

Top Aphrodisiac. YLANG YLANG is considered to be very sensual oil, euphoric and, of course, romantic. It is also considered to be soothing. In aromatherapy, it has the ability to positively impact emotions and can help create a sensual atmosphere in your home.

Natural Aphrodisiac. Used through time for this purpose, the components of CINNAMON encourage circulation and warmth. While Ylang Ylang (the other highly known aphrodisiac) is flowery and more "girly", CINNAMON is more spicy and some men prefer the scent.

Mild Aphrodisiac. NEROLI and SWEET ORANGE have aphrodisiac qualities! Create an environment in your bedroom – or make your own perfume by blending 4 drops of NEROLI into your favorite cream or oil – dot it on your body and behind your ears!

Boost Sexual Desire: CLARY SAGE is a substance or stimulus that boosts libido and feelings of sexual desire. It is very effective in treating frigidity, psychological problems resulting in loss of libido, and even impotency.

Libido. STAR ANISE is sometimes used to help increase libido in the East.

Boost Sexual Energy: Blend 4 drops CLARY SAGE, 2 drops JASMINE, 4 drops SANDALWOOD in 4 teaspoons of a carrier and massage on your pulse points and abdomen.

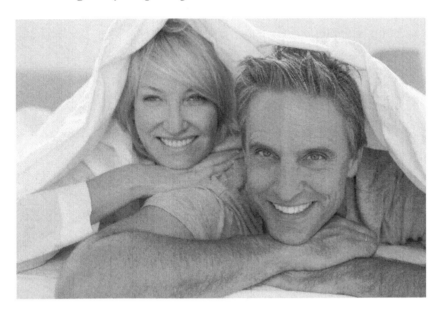

RINSE OR CLEANSE FRUIT

ESSENTIAL OILS USED IN THIS SECTION:
BERGAMOT, LEMON, CITRUS ESSENTIAL OILS

Get rid of pesticides & toxins. If you are worried about pesticides on your fresh fruit and veggies, add 2-4 drops of BERGAMOT to half a gallon of water and cleanse – then rinse!

Or use LEMON or any of the CITRUS oils.

Following a study conducted by the U.S. Department of Agriculture, using LEMON (or BERGAMOT) could help protect against such pathogens like E. coli and Salmonella.

TOILET ROOM HACK

I love this tip: Add a drop or two of BERGAMOT, ROSE GERANIUM, NEROLI or your favorite oil to the inside of your toilet paper roll (the cardboard roller). Every time you or a guest takes some toilet paper and move the roller, a little aroma is released and freshens the room!

FRESH BED MATTRESS

ESSENTIAL OILS USED IN THIS SECTION: LAVENDER OR CLARY SAGE

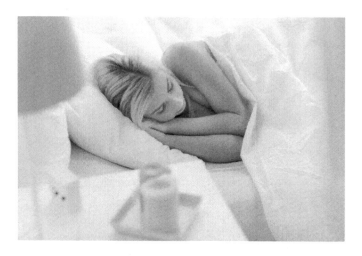

Freshen that mattress and get rid of dust mites and microbes. This is especially good if you have an older mattress and no budget to buy a new bed in the immediate future.

1) Put 1 cup of baking soda in a small mason jar, and add 5 drops of LAVENDER (or CLARY SAGE.) Shake it up well!
2) Now, strip the bed and wash your linens. Take your mixture to the mattress and lightly sprinkle the mixture into a light dusting on top of the mattress (you can use a sifter if want to control the amount.)
3) Let it sit for at least an hour (longer is better) to draw out moisture, dirt, do its antibacterial work and also give the mattress a nice lavender deodorizing.
4) When ready, vacuum your mattress until the dusting is entirely gone. Now you have a fresh mattress that is lightly scented of

LAVENDER, helpful for sleep!

Chapter 4
Home Pharmacy of Essential Oils

Here are several suggestions to create your own Home Pharmacy. We have grouped some of the most performing Essential Oils that handle a wide variety of issues together for your convenience. With either pack, your safety tips and this book, you would be ready for action, and can also speak more intelligently to a doctor, aromatherapist or holistic doctor about your needs.

You might like to listen to my Essential Oil Zen podcast episode about the Home Pharmacy!

BASIC HOME PHARMACY PACK

(6 Essential Oils: Lavender, Peppermint, Eucalyptus, Clary Sage, Lemon and Frankincense.)

HOME PHARMACY II (10 Essential Oils)

(Lavender, Peppermint, Eucalyptus, Clary Sage, Lemon, Frankincense, Cedarwood, Cinnamon, Star Anise and Immune Boost Blend)

TIME SAVERS – BLENDS READY TO GO

Many reputable companies put blend together. Some are mixed in a carrier for topical use, and some are mixed without carrier for diffusion.

My company Sublime Naturals, offers therapeutic-grade essential oils and blends, and here are our **CUSTOMER FAVORITE Ready-To-Go Blends**:

Uplift, Happiness: ZEN AIR BLISS ZEN Diffuser Blend

Purify the Air of Microbes, Create a Calming Environment: ZEN AIR SOOTHE & PURIFY Diffuser Blend

Topical to Bring Down Stress: ZEN DESTRESS Essential Oil Blend

Topical for Daily Immune Support: ZEN IMMUNE BOOST Essential Oil Blend

Diffuser Blend for Immune Support: ZEN AIR IMMUNE BOOST (small bottle)

Topical for Sore Muscles: ZEN SORE MUSCLE Essential Oil Blend

Topical for Better Sleep: Zen SUBLIME SLEEP Essential Oil Blend (+ Diffuse Lavender)

Topical for Help with Focus: ZEN FOCUS Essential Oil Blend

DOSAGE & DILUTE CHART RECOMMENDATIONS

The chart on the next page suggests how much of a dilution or dosage you or your family should consider using when using Essential Oils topically.

You will see that a 1% dilution is 5-6 drops of an essential oil in 1 ounce of your carrier. This is a recommendation for children, the ill, those with compromised immune systems and the aged.

A 2% dilution is 10-12 drops in an ounce of carrier, and this is typically suggested for massage oils and typical uses by health adults.

Now for more urgent, short-term uses, like treating congestion, a bad cough or flu, a severe headache or sprain, **a 3% to 10% dilution** is more rare and is for specific short-term issues. That is 15 to18 drops in an ounce up to 50-60 drops for 10%, for severe emergency-type cases.

Using and Essential Oil "neat", as you have learned, means putting it directly on your skin. Only a few Essential Oils qualify for this use (others are too harsh and can burn or agitate.) Using an oil "neat" is also for short term, more emergency-like situations, such as disinfecting a new cut. You typically use 1-2 drops neat.

A few of my suggestions in the book may be lower doses, but you can always add several drops more if desired.

DILUTION GUIDE

ESSENTIAL OILS

SUBLIME BEAUTY NATURALS AND ZEN BOX

1% DILUTION
5-6 drops of essential oil in 1 ounce of carrier oil

FOR CHILDREN, PREGNANT WOMAN, Those with **COMPROMISED IMMUNE SYSTEM, Use on FACE,**

2% DILUTION
10-12 drops of essential oil in 1 ounce carrier oil

FOR MASSAGE OIL, DAILY USE BY HEALTHY ADULTS

3-10% DILUTION
3%= 15-18 drops of essential oil in 1 oz carrier oil
10%=50-60 drops.

FOR SHORT-TERM SITUATIONAL USE Like Chest Congestion, injury of muscles, sprains

"NEAT"USE
Undiluted with Carrier Oil. Some Oils can be used in small areas for acute situations

SHORT-TERM LOCAL INJURY, SMALL AREAS Like Cuts, Burns, Bug Bites. Lavender and Tea Tree are 2 often used.

BIBLIOGRAPHY

Balz, Rodolphe. The Healing Power of Essential Oils. Lotus Light. 1996.

Butje, Andrea. Essential Living: Aromatherapy Recipes for Health & Home. 2nd edition. 2015.

Gattefossé, Rene-Maurice. Aromatherapy. Translated by Robert B. Tisserand. Saffron Walden, 1993.

Harding, Jennie. The Essential Oils Handbook. Watkins Publishing London. 2008.

Johnson, Dr. Scott A. Evidence-Based Essential Oil Therapy. Scott A. Johnson Professional Writing Services, LLC , 2015

Lawless, Julia. The Illustrated Encyclopedia of Essential Oils. Thorsons, 1995.

Purchon, Nerys & Cantele, Lora. The Complete Aromatherapy & Essential Oils Handbook. Robert Rose Press. 2014.

Schnaubelt, Dr. Kurt. Advanced Aromatherapy. Healing Arts Press, 1998.

Schnaubelt, Dr. Kurt. The Healing Intelligence of Essential Oils. Healing Arts Press, 2011.

Schnaubelt, Dr. Kurt. Medical Aromatherapy. Frog, Ltd. 1999.

Tisserand, Robert B. The Art of Aromatherapy. Healing Arts Press. 1977

Tisserand, Robert B. and Young, Rodney. Essential Oil Safety: A Guide for Healthcare Professionals. 2nd edition. Churchill Livingstone.

Wildwood, Chrissie. The Encyclopedia of Aromatherapy. Healing Arts Press, 2000.

Worwood, Valerie Ann. The Complete Book of Essential Oils & Aromatherapy. New World Library. 1991.

ACKNOWLEDGEMENTS

I acknowledge and thank the long-term experts and those I have learned from and am learning from, from Paris days through current days, including Robert Tisserand, Andrea Butje, David Crow, Dr. Axe and Sayer Ji. I admire them and their work! I thank the NAHA association as well.

I acknowledge and look forward to the work of Angela Jensen Ehmke and Kristina Bauer, (executive producers) of the upcoming movie "Uncommon Scents", for which I am a small contributer.

Thanks to my husband Harlan for all of his support, as always!

ABOUT THE AUTHOR

Thanks so much for reading my book. I hope it will help you and your family for years to come.

I specialize in books about wellness & beauty - with a niche in essential oils and aromatherapy! I lived in Paris, France for 16 years which greatly influenced me and my knowledge of essential oils and beauty techniques.

Visit www.BooksByHeshelow.com to get a free book! I often run gift giveaways and secret information & deals for my followers!

Some of my newest books include "Break Sugar Cravings or Addiction, Feel Full, Lose Weight: An Astonishing Essential Oil Method", "The Crisis of Antibiotic-Resistant Bacteria & How Essential Oils Help," "Essential Oils have Super Powers®", "Phytoceramides: Anti Aging at its Best" and "Turmeric: How to Use It For YOUR Wellness" or see my list on Amazon here.

THE REASON I WRITE: to help you discover new information, techniques or improve your health and wellness!

I'm a member of NAHA (National Association for Holistic Aromatherapy) and an aromatherapist certification student at Aromahead Institute. An entrepreneur, I founded and run Sublime Beauty® and Sublime Beauty Naturals® and live in the St. Petersburg, Florida area with my better-half hubby and pup.

I do hope you will write a review of this book – it means the world to authors including me to hear what you think! Do reach out with any questions!

Sincerely, Kathy Heshelow

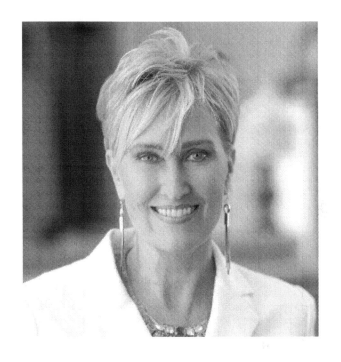

Made in the USA
Monee, IL
18 November 2019